THE TM RESEARCH SUMMARY BOOK

David Orme-Johnson PhD

Denise Denniston Gerace PhD

CONTENTS

Preface:
A Brief History of TM

Transcendental Meditation, or TM, is an effortless, easily learned technique for allowing the conscious mind to settle down and "transcend" the conscious thinking process while remaining alert and awake. The neurological, physiological, and sociological effects of regularly experiencing that inner state of silence are the subject of the research summarized here.

TM was introduced to the world by Maharishi Mahesh Yogi, whose training both in physics and traditional Vedic literature made him uniquely qualified to bridge the gap between the subjective systems of the East and the objective systems of science. His goal was simple: to ensure that any person, now or in the future, could enjoy the benefits of this knowledge.

Toward a Science of Mind

Western cultures have long sought a "science of mind," or "first science," one that goes beyond psychology to the origins and basis of human consciousness.

Eastern traditions have preserved a rich history of approaches to such a science, but the literature is often too diverse and esoteric to achieve synergy with Western approaches to knowledge.

Maharishi's approach was to present a purely systematic procedure based on a long tradition of Vedic scholars, going back hundreds (if not thousands) of years, whose experience combined both subjective and objective understanding of the mechanics of the thinking process. The Transcendental Meditation technique is the practical embodiment of that tradition. It has stood the test of time.

Practice vs Technique

Three important aspects of the TM program make it unique among all the meditative, contemplative, or other eyes-closed practices.

First and foremost, TM is not, strictly speaking, a practice: it is a *technique* analogous to the one we all use for going to sleep—we *initiate* a natural process; we don't *do* the sleeping. (The word "practice," of course, also refers to *regularly* applying the technique.)

TM aims to de-excite mental activity, leading to the experience of "pure" consciousness—silent awareness without the incessant excitation of thoughts and the complexity of the mental landscape. It should be self-evident that engaging in a practice for a period of time cannot constitute mental inactivity. Thus, a technique is required to allow the neurophysiology *to settle down of its own accord.*

Natural

Second, because the TM technique is a natural process, one that anyone can do, it is safe, harmless, and effortless, and does not rely on acceptance of a value system or belief in a world-view, and is compatible with virtually any religion or philosophy.

How TM Is Taught—Consistency and Repeatability

Third, and of greatest significance to this research summary, TM is taught in precisely the same way in every country. Teachers of TM are certified by a rigorous program that ensures the exact same procedure is followed for imparting the technique to anyone.

For people learning the TM program (TM for 20 minutes twice a day), this means that all the studies summarized here describe the exact technique they are learning. All the findings of the TM research in this book will, in some measure, apply to them.

For scientists studying TM and the TM program, this uniformity of methodology ensures maximum repeatability of experimental results. This consistency of the program among all TMers is rarely found in other eyes-closed practices.

About this Book

This book is a condensation of the research presented in *The TM & TM-Sidhi Book*, a comprehensive introduction to the TM technique, the TM program, and several related programs introduced by Maharishi that are based on other long-standing Indian traditions. The TM-Sidhi program is an advanced variant of the TM technique; the related programs represent new directions for research and experience in psychology, architecture, medicine & health, and the arts. These expansions, based on the TM program, may best be explored in the courses offered at MIU (Maharishi International University).

Dedication

All the books in the "TM Book" series are dedicated to Maharishi and the Vedic tradition of teachers whom he represented, and to Tony Nader, MD, PhD, MARR, the global Head of the Transcendental Meditation organization. Dr. Nader trained in medicine at Harvard University and received his PhD in neuroscience at Massachusetts Institute of Technology. He is also a globally recognized Vedic scholar, trained and appointed by Maharishi as his successor. He explains how consciousness structures the world, and how we can take advantage of that, in his book, *Consciousness Is All there Is.*

Other Peer-Reviewed Research

Please see MIU.edu, TM.org, and TruthAboutTM.org for more information.

— Allen Cobb, Editor

Meditations Differ in How Much Effort They Require & Their Effects on the EEG Frequency

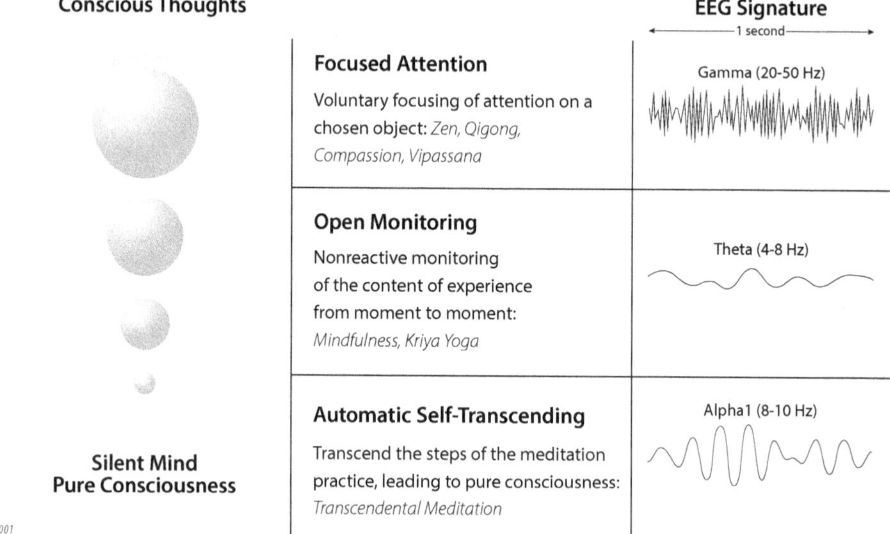

Diagram Reference: Travis, F.T., & Shear, J. (2010). Focused attention, open monitoring and automatic self-transcending: Categories to organize meditations from Vedic, Buddhist and Chinese traditions. *Consciousness and Cognition*, 19(4), 1110–1118.

DIFFERENT MEDITATIONS WORK DIFFERENTLY

Focused Attention

These techniques involve concentrating or focusing on something—a word, an idea, a goal—or just making the mind blank. The high-frequency gamma EEG associated with focused attention is believed to bind together spatially close cortical areas needed for sharply focusing attention outward, such as to a novel experience.

Open Monitoring

Open Monitoring, such as mindfulness, asks the person to notice what is happening without getting involved. Theta EEG is believed to reflect inhibition of outer sensory information that might disturb the person's inner thought processes, such as when they are monitoring their subjective experiences.

Spontaneous Self-Transcending

The Transcendental Meditation (TM) technique allows the mind to actually settle down, to pause in its more active ways of working and just be awake and aware. It is an effortless process that is associated with Alpha1 EEG, a state of restful alertness. During this profound state of deep rest, the whole brain works together, which science calls coherence. This deep rest and the brain working together are two "active ingredients" in TM that account for the much greater changes that TM produces in the mind and body on important things like anxiety, blood pressure, and overall health.

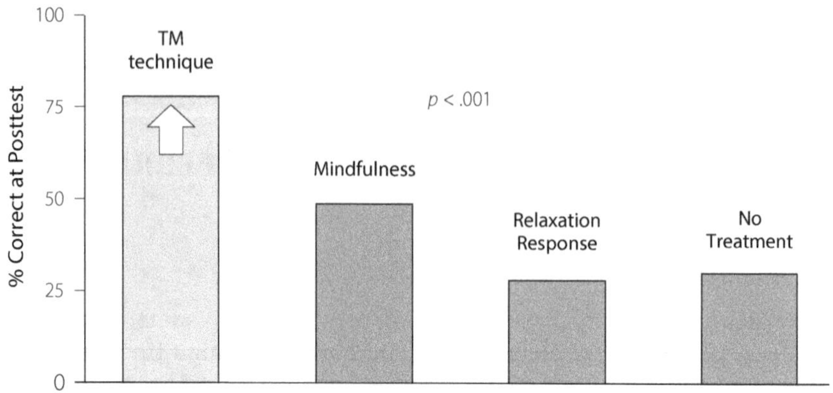

A study of 80-year-olds conducted at Harvard found that practice of TM increases cognitive flexibility.

tm-002

TM WORKS BETTER

Researchers have found a marked decline in cognitive functioning with advancing age. Research on the Transcendental Meditation (TM) program has shown it to be a great tool for improving cognitive flexibility and memory in elders.

A study of 80-year-olds, conducted at Harvard and published in the prestigious *Journal of Personality and Social Psychology*, found that the practice of the Transcendental Meditation technique increases cognitive flexibility. Cognitive flexibility was measured by the ability to learn new material that was different from previously learned material, that is, the ability to overcome old habits with new knowledge. (Reference 1)

The study also found that TM practice reduced systolic blood pressure more than the other techniques.

Practicing TM was shown to extend life, with a higher quality of life. At the three-year followup, 100% of the TMers were still alive, whereas only 63% to 87% of the other groups (elders practicing mindfulness, relaxation, or no treatment) were still alive.

Other studies have shown higher levels of cognitive functioning and lower levels of free radicals (lipid peroxide) in elders who practice TM. (Reference 2)

Reference 1: Alexander, C.N., Langer, E.J., Newman, R.I., et al. Transcendental Meditation, mindfulness, and longevity: an experimental study with the elderly. *Journal of Personality and Social Psychology* 57, no. 6 (1989): 950–964.

Reference 2: Nidich, S.I., Schneider, R.H., Nidich, R.J., Foster, G., Sharma, H., Salerno, J.W., ..., Alexander, C.N. (2005). Effect of the Transcendental Meditation program on intellectual development in community-dwelling older adults. *Journal of Social Behavior and Personality*, 17(1), 217–228.

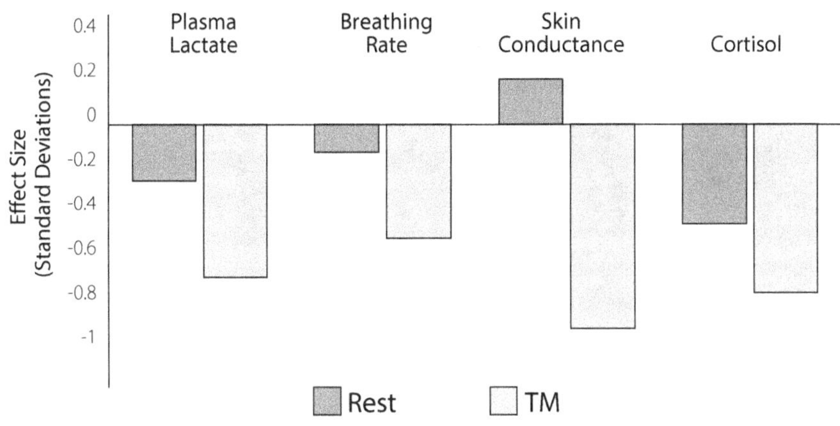

PROFOUND DEEP REST AT WILL

This chart shows a synthesis (a meta-analysis) of all the research done on changes in stress indicators (32 studies) during the Transcendental Meditation (TM) technique. It confirms that the state achieved during TM is profoundly relaxing, as indicated by the following physiological changes:

- decreased plasma lactate (a metabolic byproduct), which indicates rejuvenation of the body

- decreased breathing rate, which indicates a more relaxed physiology

- decreased skin conductance, as seen from less sweaty palms, which indicates that stress is decreasing

- decreased cortisol, the major stress hormone, which indicates a holistic reduction in the stress response

These physiological changes correspond to the changes in brain activity during TM practice and to the increases in EEG coherence.

References: Dillbeck, M.C., Orme-Johnson, D.W. Physiological differences between Transcendental Meditation and rest. *American Psychologist.* 1987;42:879–81.

Jevning, R., Wilson, A.F., Davidson, J.M. Adrenocortical activity during meditation. *Hormones and Behavior* 10, no. 1 (1978): 54–60.

Michaels R.R., Parra, J., McCann, D.S., Vander, A.J. Renin, Cortisol, and Aldosterone During Transcendental Meditation. *Psychosomatic Medicine* 1979;41(1):50–54.

Also see Klimes-Dougan, B., Shen, C.L., Samikoglu, A., Thai, M., Amatya, P., Cullen, K.R., & Lim, K.O. (2019). Transcendental Meditation and Hypothalamic-Pituitary-Adrenal Axis functioning: A pilot, randomized controlled trial with young adults. *Stress: The International Journal on the Biology of Stress.*

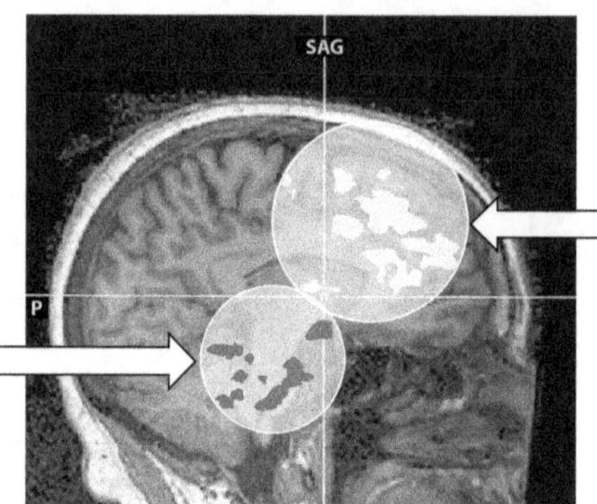

PROFOUND REST & SETTLED AWARENESS

This study used a brain imaging technique called functional Magnetic Resonance Imaging (fMRI), which shows which areas of the brain increase (light) or decrease (dark) in blood flow, which indicates the increase or decrease in activity in different areas of the brain.

The pattern of blood flow during Transcendental Meditation (TM) practice indicates a state of Restful Alertness. During TM, we are seeing increased blood flow (light) in the executive frontal cortical brain areas, which correlates with increased inner awareness during TM. At the same time we see brain changes associated with deep relaxation, as indicated by reduced activity in the brainstem and cerebellum shown in the circled dark areas. Reduced activity in the brainstem is associated with slower breathing, reduced heart rate, and decreased blood pressure, if it is too high. The cerebellum is generally understood as governing muscle tone, balance, and coordination of motor activity. Decreased activity in this area corresponds to a deeply relaxed body during TM practice.

We see in this that TM is simultaneously affecting the brain on its most basic level (brainstem) and its highest level, the frontal "Chief Executive Officer" of the brain. This is different from what we see in drowsiness and sleep, where frontal blood flow decreases, corresponding to the loss of awareness. Also, other meditation techniques do not produce this pattern. Thus, TM produces a unique state of restful alertness that has proven highly beneficial for allowing the body's self-repair mechanisms to efficiently normalize stresses in the physiology.

Reference: Mahone, M.C., Travis, F., Gevirtz, R., & Hubbard, D. (2018). fMRI during Transcendental Meditation practice. *Brain and Cognition*, Epub 2018 Mar 2.

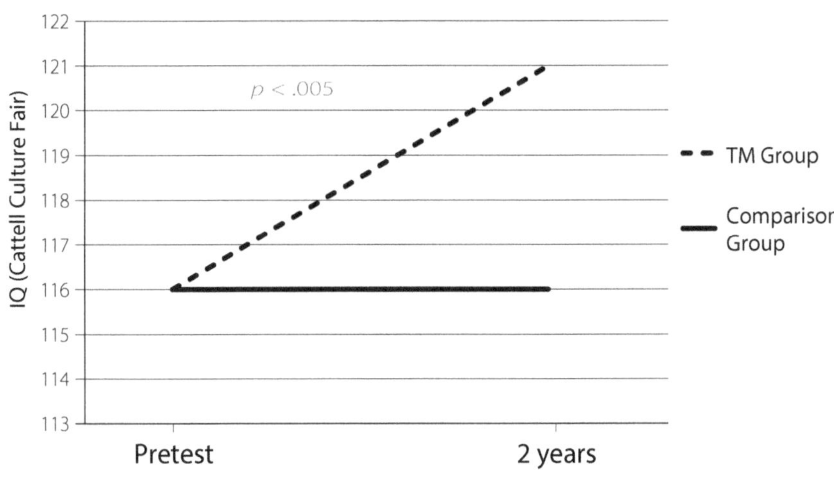

INCREASING INTELLIGENCE

Fluid intelligence is the ability to come up with solutions in novel situations for which there is no prior learning or manual on what to do. Research has shown that fluid intelligence increases up until adolescence, then is believed not to increase further. There have been many attempts to increase it in the history of psychology and nothing has worked—until several studies on the Transcendental Meditation (TM) program have shown that it is possible.

This two-year study found an unprecedented growth in fluid intelligence by five IQ points in college students practicing TM. Control subjects who received only the usual college curriculum and not TM training did not change.

The students were an average of 25 years old, an age at which fluid intelligence is not expected to increase. Control subjects who received only the usual college curriculum and not TM training did not change on fluid intelligence, as was expected for their age group. (Reference 1) Two additional studies found that TM increases fluid intelligence in college students. (Reference 2) TM has also been found to increase fluid intelligence in high school students. (Reference 3)

Reference 1: Cranson, R.W., Orme-Johnson, D.W., Gackenbach, J., Dillbeck, M.C., Jones, C.H., Alexander, C.N. Transcendental Meditation and improved performance on intelligence-related measures: a longitudinal study. *Personality and Individual Differences*. 1991;12:1105–16.

Reference 2: Dillbeck, M.C., Raimondi, D., Assimakis, P.D., Rowe, R., & Orme-Johnson, D.W. (1986). Longitudinal effects of the Transcendental Meditation and TM-Sidhi program on cognitive ability and cognitive style. *Perceptual and Motor Skills*, 62(731–738).

Reference 3: So, K.T., Orme-Johnson, D.W. Three randomized experiments on the holistic longitudinal effects of the Transcendental Meditation technique on cognition. *Intelligence* 29, no. 5 (2001): 419–440.

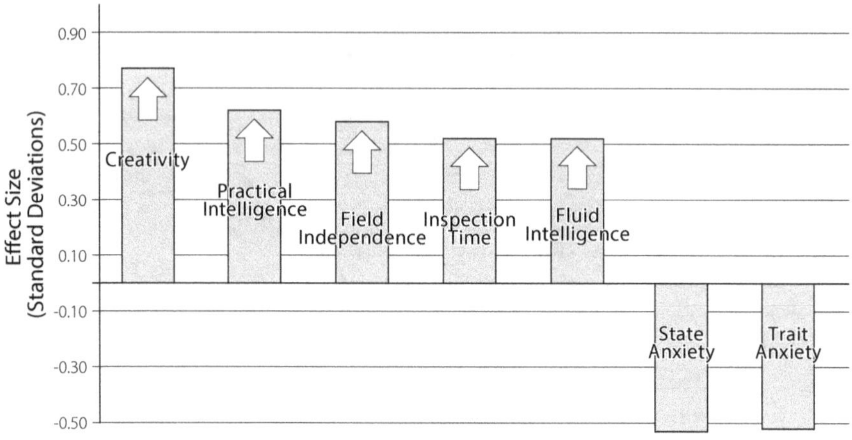

INCREASED INTELLIGENCE, LESS STRESS & ANXIETY

Three studies on the Transcendental Meditation (TM) program were conducted in high schools, two of the studies over a period of six months and the third one for a year. Students were randomly assigned to practice TM or to be in one of three comparison groups in which the students either: 1) napped, 2) practiced another meditation technique, or 3) just had school as usual with no treatment. The chart above shows changes in the TM students compared to other treatments for the three studies combined. TM produced highly significant improvements on all variables (p's < .001) compared to comparison groups. The meaning of the different measures is described below.

- **Creativity** measured "whole-brained creativity," which requires intelligent thinking on the basis of balanced emotions.

- **Practical Intelligence** measured nonintellectual abilities and attitudes that predict success in work, love, and social relationships. Increased practical intelligence helps one achieve and maintain emotional and physical wellbeing.

- **Field Independence** reflects broad comprehension with the ability to remain focused in an environment of confusion. People who are more field independent are better able to see other people's perspectives, more able to organize their thoughts, and are less influenced by social pressure.

- **Inspection Time** is a computerized test of speed of decision-making in a complex situation. It is correlated with fluid intelligence.

- **Fluid Intelligence** is the ability to find solutions in novel situations for which prior education ("book learning") does not prepare one.

- **State Anxiety** is how anxious one is at the current moment.

- **Trait Anxiety** is how anxious one is in general.

Reference: So, K.T., Orme-Johnson D.W. Three randomized experiments on the holistic longitudinal effects of the Transcendental Meditation technique on cognition. *Intelligence* 29, no. 5 (2001): 419–440.

Improved Academic Performance

Increased Math Achievement
in Students Below Proficiency
p = .001

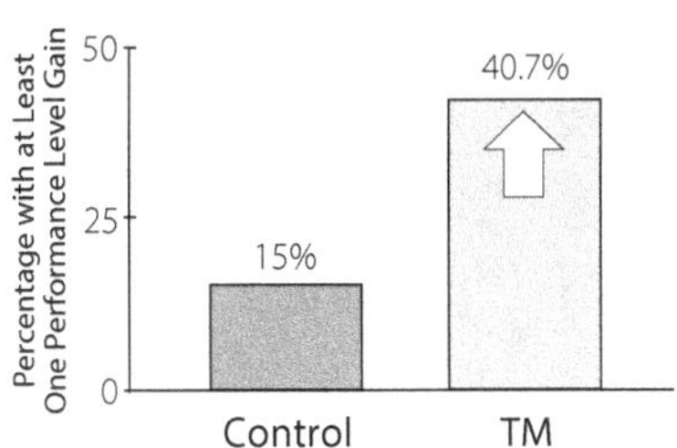

Increased English Achievement
in Students Below Proficiency
p = .005

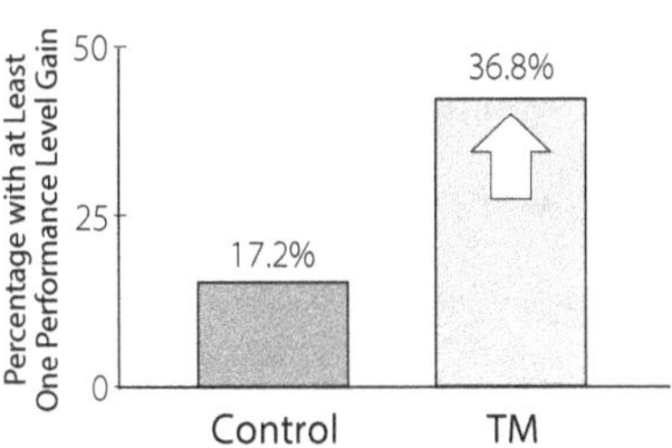

tm-007

DO BETTER IN MATH & LANGUAGE

Middle schools are of particular concern to educators because of students' poor performance on standardized tests, which predicts poor performance in further education and less success in life.

This study evaluated change in academic achievement in public middle school students practicing the Transcendental Meditation (TM) program compared to controls. A total of 189 students who were below proficiency level at baseline in English and math were evaluated for change in academic achievement using the California Standards Tests (CST). All students were from the same school and continued with the school's standard curriculum and instruction. Ninety-seven percent were racial and ethnic minority students.

TM was practiced at school twice a day as part of the school's Quiet Time program for three months prior to post-testing. Results indicated improvement for TM students compared to controls on English scale scores (p = .002) and math scale scores (p < .001). A greater percentage of TM students improved at least one performance level in math and English compared to controls (p values < .01).

P values, or probability, show the likelihood that the results were due to chance. P < .001 means that there is less than one chance in a thousand that the results were due to chance. That is, the result appears to be a true effect of TM and not some other random factor.

Reference: Nidich, S., Mjasiri, S., Nidich, N., Rainforth, M., Grant, J., Valosek, L., ..., Zigler, R.L. (2011). Academic achievement and transcendental meditation: a study with at-risk urban middle school students. *Education*, 131(3), 556–564.

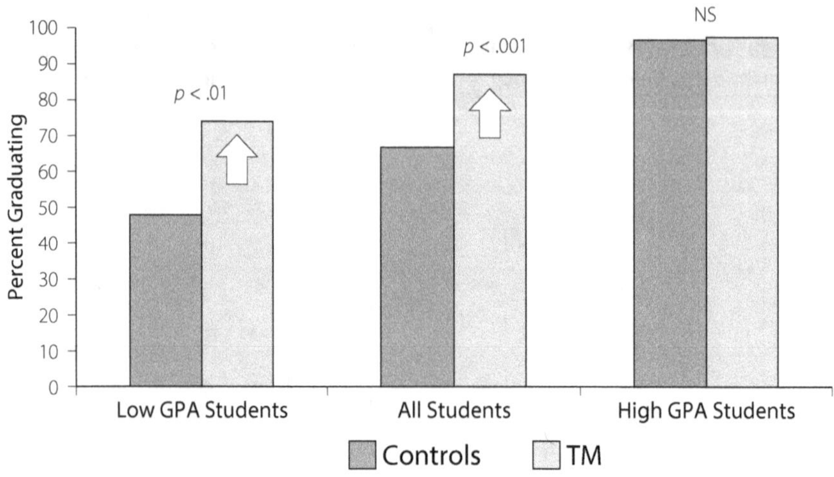

MORE SUCCESS IN SCHOOL

Practice of the Transcendental Meditation (TM) technique increased the percentage of high school students graduating, especially those with low grade point averages.

National high school graduation rates have declined in recent years, despite public and private efforts. The purpose of the current study was to determine whether students practicing the Quiet Time / TM program at a medium-size urban school had higher school graduation rates, compared to students who did not receive training in this stress-reduction program.

An analysis, based on school records, was conducted on all 235 students enrolled during their senior year. Overall the percentage of TM students graduating was 87.1% and the percentage of non-meditating students graduating was only 66.7% (p <.001). Results from a matched controlled subgroup indicated that for the low GPA students, 72.9% of the TM students graduated compared to only 47.9% of the non-meditating students (p = .012).

Significant differences were also found for dropout rates and college acceptance.

These results indicate that TM is a viable program for increasing graduation rates in urban schools.

Reference: Colbert, R.D., & Nidich, S. (2013). Effect of the Transcendental Meditation program on graduation, college acceptance and dropout rates for students attending an urban public high school. *Education*, 133(4), 495–501.

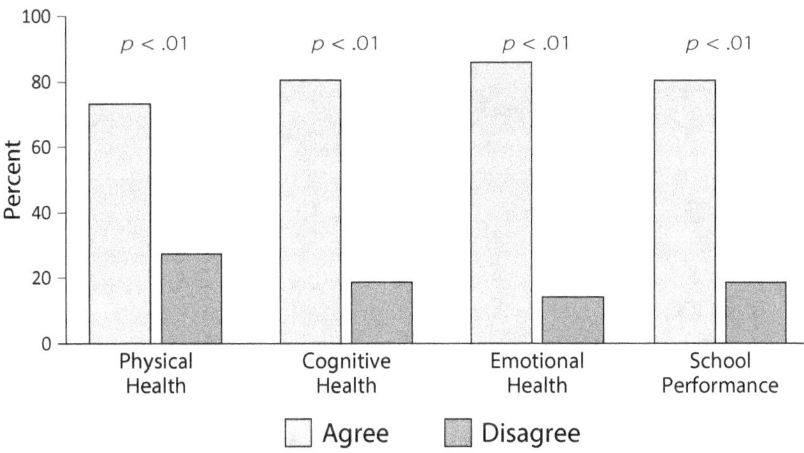

BETTER EQUIPPED FOR A GOOD LIFE

In Huay-Huay, a remote Peruvian town in the Andean mountains, in a school where all the children had learned TM, 91 randomly-selected children, ranging in age from 11 to 16 years, were given a questionnaire about their experiences with TM in four categories: physical health (more energy, better quality of sleep, good athletic ability), cognitive health (better memory, comprehension, problem-solving ability), emotional health (less aggression, friendlier, happier), and school performance (satisfaction and efficiency at school, getting along with classmates, academic achievement and learning, less truancy).

A majority of these children reported benefits across all measures, and these benefits were apparently stronger when students practiced meditation more regularly. Gender and grade level did not appear to influence this outcome. (Reference 1)

A second study used the same measure with 520 primary and secondary students at four schools in Lima, Cusco, Puno, and Ventanilla, and found similar results. (Reference 2)

In Peru, as of 2023, more than 60,000 young people, including indigenous students in remote locations, practice TM twice daily in school. Most of these are Catholic schools, in this predominantly Catholic country. This paper was published by the Education Department of the largest university in Peru, Pontificia Universidad Católica del Perú.

Reference 1: Fergusson, L., Ortiz Cabrejos, J., & Bonshek, A. (2021, September). Health and school performance: an exploratory quantitative study of school children in Huay-Huay, perú. *Educación*, *30*(59), 65.

Reference 2: Fergusson, L., Ortiz Cabrejos, J., & Bonshek, A. (2022). Meditation practice by primary and secondary students in Perú: a confirmatory study of health and school performance. *Revista Innova Educación*, *4*(1), 21-38.

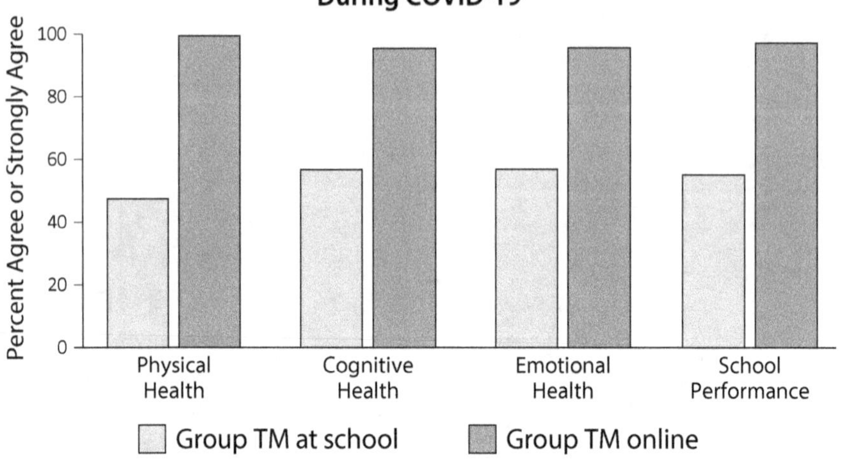

SYNCHRONIZED TM IS HIGHLY EFFECTIVE

During the COVID-19 pandemic, a study of 107 Peruvian secondary students (ages 12-16) compared those doing group practice of Transcendental Meditation (TM) while at school, with those doing group practice of TM coordinated online for students who were isolated at home.

Students rated both group TM at school and group TM from home (connected online) as being beneficial. Ratings of TM benefits from remotely-organized group TM sessions were higher, perhaps because students felt more at ease and comforted at home, were less distracted, or had a greater appreciation of the group during isolation.

In both conditions, the majority of the students rated TM to be beneficial or highly beneficial for improving physical health (more energy, better quality of sleep, and good athletic ability), cognitive health (better memory, comprehension, and problem-solving ability), emotional health (less aggression, friendlier, and happier), and school performance (satisfaction and efficiency at school, getting along with classmates, academic achievement and learning, and less truancy).

Reference: Fergusson, L., Ortiz Cabrejos, J., & Bonshek, A. (2022). Health and school performance during home isolation at Institución Educativa Privada Prescott in Puno, Perú. *Tapuya: Latin American Science, Technology and Society, 5*(1), 2003004.

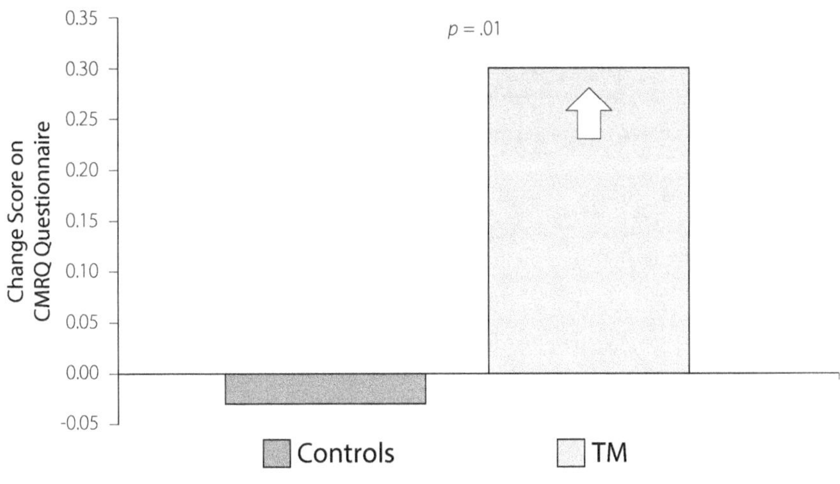

IMPROVED JOB PERFORMANCE

This three-month study evaluated the effects of the Transcendental Meditation (TM) technique on stress reduction, health, and employee development in two settings in the automotive industry: a large manufacturing plant of a Fortune 100 corporation, and a small distribution sales company, using the Center for Management Research Questionnaire (CMRQ). Employees who learned TM were compared to controls similar in worksite, job position, demographic, and pre-test characteristics.

Those who practiced TM regularly improved significantly more than controls (with irregular TMers scoring in between) on multiple measures of stress and employee development, including: reduced physiological arousal (measured by skin conductance levels) during and outside TM practice; decreased trait anxiety, job tension, insomnia and fatigue, decreased cigarette and hard liquor use; improved general health (and fewer health complaints); and enhanced employee effectiveness, job satisfaction, and work/personal relationships.

Three factors underlying this wide range of improvements through TM were: "occupational coherence," "physiological settledness," and "job and life satisfaction." The effectiveness of TM on these factors was substantially larger than for other forms of meditation and relaxation reported in four previous statistical meta-analyses.

Reference: Alexander, C.N., Swanson, G.C., Rainforth, M.V., Carlisle, T.W., Todd, C.C., Oates, R.M. Effects of the Transcendental Meditation program on stress reduction, health, and employee development: A prospective study in two occupational settings. *Anxiety, Stress and Coping: An International Journal.* 1993;6:245–62.

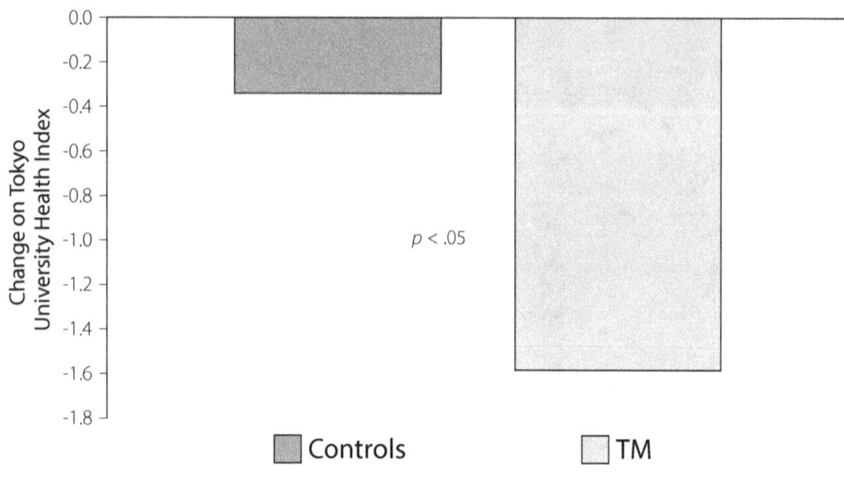

tm-012

IMPROVED SELF-CONTROL

A study conducted at Sumitomo Heavy Industries by the Japanese National Institute of Industrial Health found decreased impulsiveness in workers who learned the Transcendental Meditation (TM) program compared to non-meditating workers, who served as control subjects.

The purpose of this study was to verify the effects of TM on the health of employees in an industrial work setting. A health survey was mailed to the subjects before and after implementation of the program. 447 workers learned TM and were compared with 321 who did not learn the practice.

The study found that those who practiced TM compared to controls had:

- Fewer physical complaints
- Fewer digestive problems
- Decreased impulsiveness
- Greater emotional stability
- Decreased tendency of neurosis
- Decreased insomnia
- Decreased smoking

The findings of this study provide evidence that TM can be effectively implemented in an industrial company, with great benefits for the mental and physical health of its employees.

References: Haratani, T. & Hemmi, T. (1990). Effects of Transcendental Meditation on the mental health of industrial workers. *Japanese Journal of Industrial Health*, 32, 656.

Haratani, T. & Hemmi, T. (1990). Effects of Transcendental Meditation on health behavior of industrial workers. *Japanese Journal of Public Health*, 37(10 Suppl.), 729.

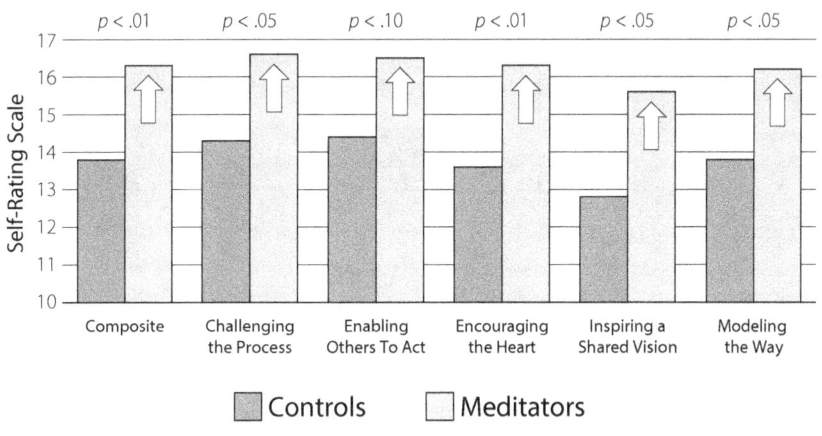

BETTER LEADERS INCREASE PRODUCTIVITY

This study was conducted at an international company in the wholesale food industry. It approached increasing productivity by improving leadership through a self-development program to strengthen the person from within. The self-development program used was the Transcendental Meditation (TM) technique, because it is known to decrease stress and increase creativity. TM subjects and non-meditating control subjects were measured on leadership behaviors before and after 4 months, and later 8 months, of TM practice.

The TM subjects improved significantly compared to controls on all leadership behaviors. They became more innovative in their thinking, challenging existing processes with "out of the box" original ideas. They became more helpful and likely to enable others to act. They began to encourage fellow employees by using "heart values" to motivate them. They inspired others to act with the shared vision of the company's goals, and they increasingly became models of ideal employees and supervisors.

Almost everyone interviewed during the program a year and a half later commented that the company as a whole was much more upbeat and that employees were more rested and were enjoying work. An outside observer said all the employees seemed more on top of their work, much less in crisis mode. From a business angle, the company reached highs in quarterly sales.

Reference: McCollum, B. (1999). Leadership development and self development: an empirical study. *Career Development International*, 4(3), 149–154.

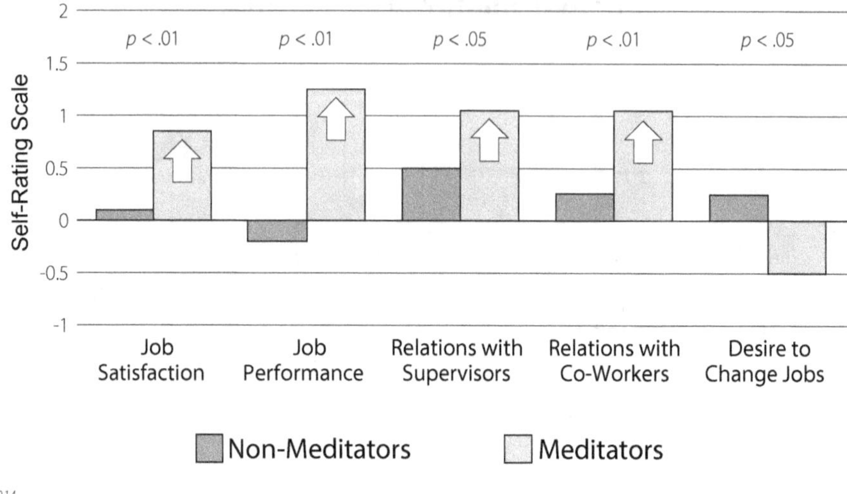

MORE JOB SUCCESS

This is a study of how the Transcendental Meditation (TM) technique affected the work experience of TMers in their primary work organization compared to non-TMers. The study found that TM significantly improves job satisfaction, job performance, and relations with supervisors and co-workers. TMers also felt more satisfaction with their work environments, as indicated by decreased desire to change jobs.

At every level of organization, performance improved when the members practiced TM. Within the organizational structure, TMers succeeded more quickly and experienced less anxiety. Their fellow employees saw them as moving ahead quickly. This indicates that a faster pace of progress is natural for a person practicing the Transcendental Meditation technique.

Reference: Frew, D.R. (1974/2017). Transcendental Meditation and Productivity. *Academy of Management Journal*, 17(2), 362–368.

Increased Autonomic Stability

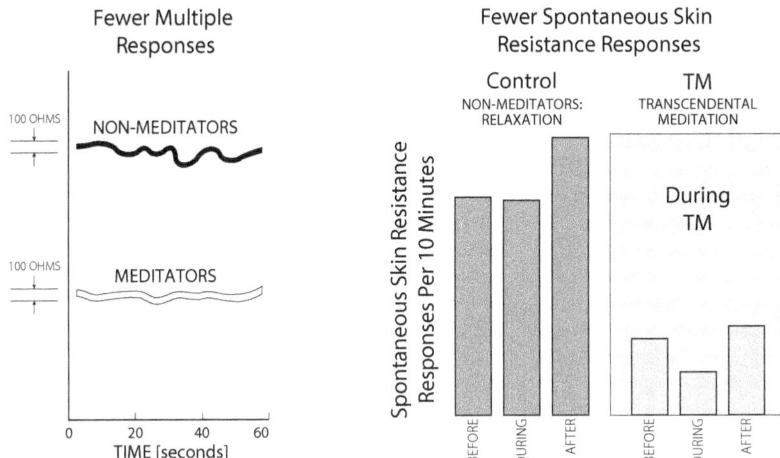

MORE STABLE UNDER PRESSURE

This landmark study conducted in the early 1970s provided physiological evidence for the first time in history that meditation of any kind could make a person feel less stressed and live a calmer lifestyle. The world is as we are—a stressed person experiences the world more stressfully than a calm person. Sometimes we find ourselves in a stressful situation we cannot change. But we can change ourselves and how we react to stress. This is what this chart on the Transcendental Meditation (TM) technique and autonomic stability shows.

The study measured slight changes in skin resistance, small stress responses, reflecting mini-changes in sweat on the palms of the hand while the subjects were sitting in a quiet room. They are called spontaneous responses because they occur without anything happening in the environment. They reflect how much stress the person is carrying around within them.

The left side of the chart above compares typical recordings from non-TMers and TMers. The non-TMers had more wavy traces, indicating more spontaneous skin resistance responses (stresses) than the TMers. The bar charts on the right show that the number of spontaneous skin resistance responses was higher for the control group than for the TM group, which had fewer spontaneous skin responses before, during, and after TM, with the greatest reduction during meditation, indicating that it is a relaxed state of stress reduction.

In two other experiments, TMers were found to make fewer spontaneous skin responses than control subjects, both during meditation and while out of meditation with eyes open.

This study also found that the TMers recovered faster from stressfully loud tones. When people carry less stress around in them, as shown in this chart, they react more calmly to stressors. A meta-analysis has found that these results have been replicated many times.

Reference: Orme-Johnson, D.W. Autonomic stability and Transcendental Meditation. *Psychosomatic Medicine* 1973 35(4):341–349

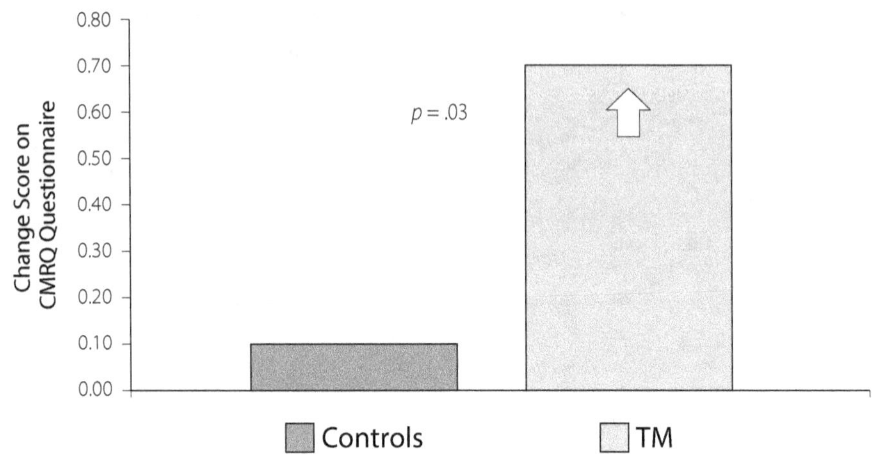

MORE SATISFIED WITH LIFE

A study of executives and workers in the automotive industry, using the Center for Management Research Questionnaire (CMRQ), found that after three months of regular practice of the Transcendental Meditation (TM) technique, participants showed increased professional and personal satisfaction, in comparison to controls from the same work sites. (Reference 1)

A related study found that TM significantly increases emotional intelligence and reduces perceived stress in administrators working in the central offices of the San Francisco Unified School District who were interested as part of a workplace wellness program. Emotional intelligence refers to the ability to perceive emotions in oneself and others, and to understand, regulate, and use such information in productive ways that lead to successful problem solving and progress of the organization as a whole toward its goals.

This study also found significant improvements in general mood, stress management, adaptability, and intrapersonal awareness. Importantly, compliance with TM practice was high (93%). (Reference 2)

These findings indicate effectiveness of implementing the TM program as a workplace wellness program to improve emotional intelligence and reduce perceived stress in employees.

Reference 1: Alexander, C.N., Swanson, G.C., Rainforth, M.V., Carlisle, T.W., Todd, C.C., & Oates, R.M. (1993). Effects of the Transcendental Meditation program on stress reduction, health, and employee development: A prospective study in two occupational settings. *Anxiety, Stress and Coping: An International Journal*, 6, 245–262.

Reference 2: Valosek, L., Link, J., Mills, P., Konrad, A., Rainforth, M., & Nidich, S. (2018). Effect of meditation on emotional intelligence and perceived stress in the workplace: A randomized controlled study. *The Permanente Journal* (E-pub: 10/29/2018).

Improved Work and Personal Relationships

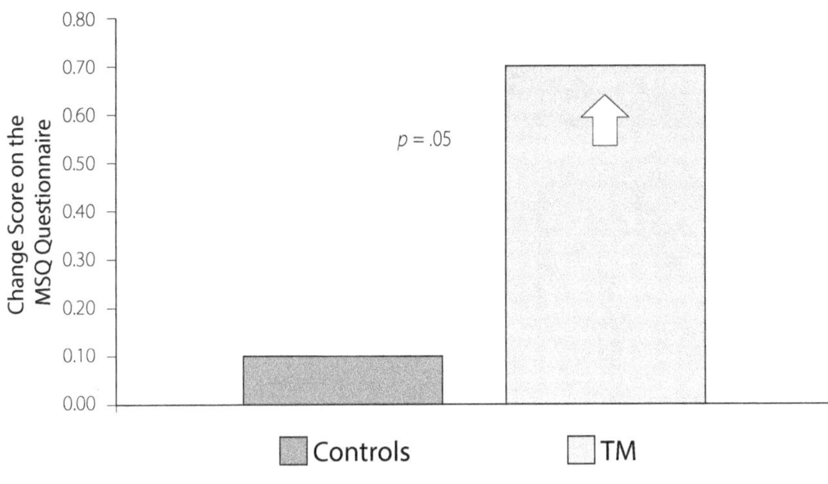

GET ALONG BETTER AT HOME & AT WORK

A study of executives and workers in the automotive industry, using the Minnesota Satisfaction Questionnaire (MSQ), found that after three months of regular practice of the Transcendental Meditation (TM) technique, participants showed improved work and personal relationships in comparison to controls from the same work sites. (Reference 1)

A related study of school administrators found that in four months, those who learned TM significantly increased in self-regard, emotional self-awareness, interpersonal relationships, stress tolerance, optimism, happiness, and self-actualization compared to a control group waiting to learn. (Reference 2)

These results are in accord with a meta-analysis of 42 studies that found TM to increase self-actualization more than other meditation and relaxation techniques. (Reference 3)

Another meta-analysis of 18 studies on 772 subjects found TM has significantly larger effects than mindfulness or other meditation techniques on reducing negative emotions, trait anxiety, and neuroticism, and on increasing self-realization. (Reference 4)

Reference 1: Alexander, C.N., Swanson, G.C., Rainforth, M.V., Carlisle, T.W., Todd, C.C., & Oates, R.M. (1993). Effects of the Transcendental Meditation program on stress reduction, health, and employee development: A prospective study in two occupational settings. *Anxiety, Stress and Coping: An International Journal*, 6, 245–262.

Reference 2: Valosek, L., Nidich, S., Wendt, S., Grant, J., & Nidich, R. (2019). Effect of meditation on social-emotional learning in middle school students. *Education*, 139(3), 111–119.

Reference 3: Alexander, C.N., Rainforth, M.V., & Gelderloos, P. (1991). Transcendental Meditation, Self-Actualization and Psychological Health: A Conceptual Overview and Statistical Meta-Analysis. *Journal of Social Behavior and Personality*, 6(5), 189–247.

Reference 4: Sedlmeier, P., Eberth, J., Schwarz, M., Zimmermann, D., & Haarig, F. (2012). The psychological effects of meditation: A meta-analysis. *Psychological Bulletin*, 138(6), 1139–1171.

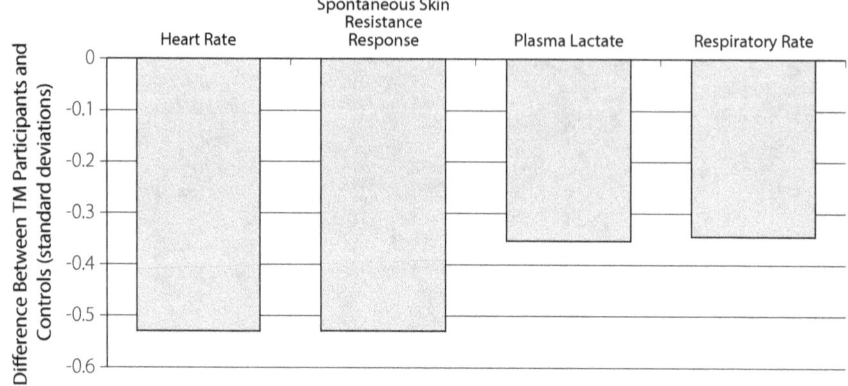

CALMER BODY & MIND

This meta-analysis of 32 studies found that Transcendental Meditation (TM) practice cultures a calmer style of physiological functioning outside of meditation, as indicated by lower levels of heart rate, spontaneous skin resistance responses, plasma lactate, and respiratory rate. (Reference 1) Living a more relaxed life is good for the heart and reduces aging, as well as reducing the risk for all types of disease.

Reduced cortisol. TM practice reduces the level of the major stress hormone cortisol in the morning for a more relaxed start of the day. (Reference 2)

Reduced teacher burnout. A randomized controlled study of secondary school teachers in Vermont, USA, found that TM significantly reduced depression, perceived stress, and overall teacher burnout. (Reference 3)

Decreased mood disturbance in family caregivers. Two months of regular practice of the Transcendental Meditation technique reduced caregivers' anxiety by 31%, depression by 31%, anger by 36%, confusion by 19%, and fatigue by 29% as compared to controls. (Reference 4)

Reference 1: Dillbeck, M.C., & Orme-Johnson, D.W. (1987). Physiological differences between Transcendental Meditation and rest. *American Psychologist*, 42, 879–881.

Reference 2: Klimes-Dougan, B., Shen C.L., Samikoglu, A., Thai, M., Amatya, P., Cullen, K.R., & Lim, K.O. (2019). Transcendental Meditation and Hypothalamic-Pituitary-Adrenal Axis functioning: A pilot, randomized controlled trial with young adults. *Stress: The International Journal on the Biology of Stress*.

Reference 3: Elder, C., Nidich, S., Moriarty, F., & Nidich, R. (2014). Effect of Transcendental Meditation on employee stress, depression, and burnout: A randomized controlled study. *The Permanente Journal*, 18(1), 19–23.

Reference 4: Nidich S., Nidich R.J., Salerno J., Hadfield B., Elder C. Stress reduction with the Transcendental Meditation program in caregivers: A pilot study. *International Archives of Nursing and Health Care Perspectives*, 2015;1(011):1–4.

Improved Hearing and Faster Reactions

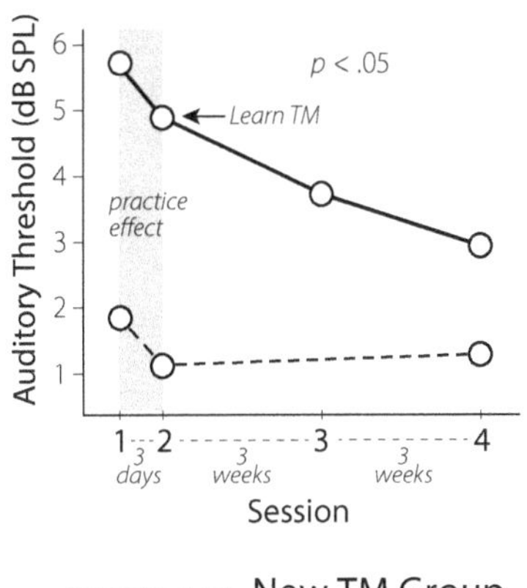

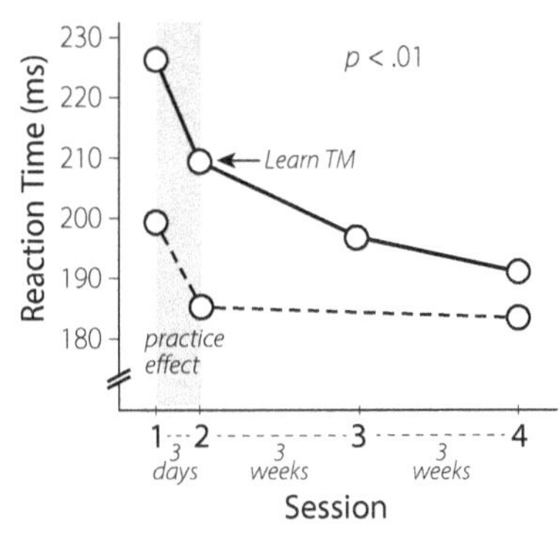

——— New TM Group   ·········· Long-Term TM Group

tm-018

HEAR BETTER, UNDERSTAND MORE

Hearing is a complex process with many stages. These studies used standard hearing tests as well as measuring multiple aspects of auditory processing in the brain. They document that TM practice improves the ability to hear, while decreasing the time it takes the brain to understand what has been heard, and to respond.

The charts above show that both the before-TM group and the long-term TM group did better on the second test, due to familiarity with the test. Three weeks after learning TM, the new TMers heard quieter things and responded to them more quickly. After six weeks of TM practice, the new TM group improved even more, on both reaction time (p<.01) and auditory thresholds (p<.05). (Reference 1)

References 2, 3, and 4 show that TM practice has a beneficial effect on processing sound from purely physical stimuli into something meaningful, including more efficient synaptic transfer, more efficient auditory pathways, greater alertness, and lower hearing threshold with TM—TMers more rapidly understand what they are hearing.

Reference 1: Schwartz, E. (1989). The effects of the Transcendental Meditation program on strength of the nervous system, perceptual reactance, reaction time, and auditory threshold. In *Scientific research on Maharishi's Transcendental Meditation and TM-Sidhi program: Collected papers* (Vol. 4, pp. 2317-2341). Maharishi Vedic University Press.

Reference 2: McEvoy, T.M., Frumpkin, L.R., & Harkins, S.W. (1980). Effects of meditation on brainstem auditory evoked potentials. *International Journal of Neuroscience*, 10(2-3), 165-170.

Reference 3: Wandhofer, A., Kobal, G., & Plattig, K.H. (1976). Shortening of latencies of human auditory evoked potentials during the Transcendental Meditation technique. *Zeitchrift fur Elektroenzephalographie und Elektromyographie EEG-EMG*, 7, 99-103.

Reference 4: Cranson, R., Goddard, P., Orme-Johnson, D.W., & Schuster, D. (1990). P300 under conditions of temporal uncertainty and filter attenuation: Reduced latency in long-term practitioners of TM. *Psychophysiology 27 27* (Suppl. 4A), S23 (Abstract).

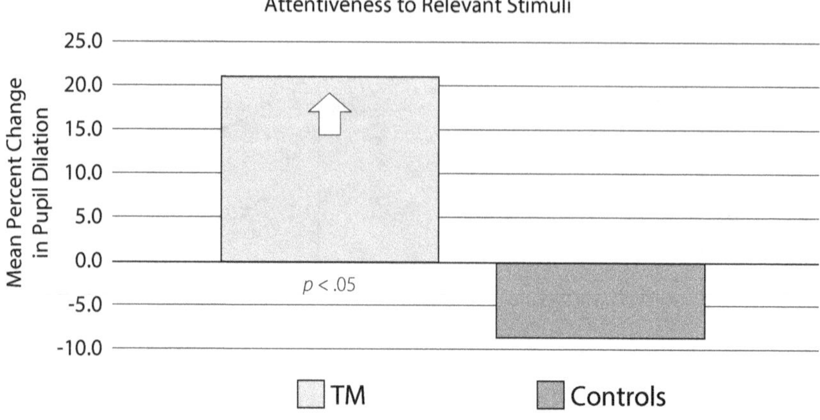

SPONTANEOUS ALERTNESS TO WHAT'S IMPORTANT

Situation awareness (SA) is the ability to know what is going on around you so that you know what to do. It is central to professions that require skill in real-time, dynamic decision-making under stress—situations characterized by high uncertainty, incomplete information, and high stakes. High-stakes professions, for example military, law enforcement, aviation and aerospace, healthcare, firefighting, self-defense, and sports, require training to maintain situation awareness to avoid costly errors in judgment. Impaired judgment and decision-making due to loss of SA in these professions can result in major loss, even loss of life.

Attentiveness is the amount of information taken in. In this study it was measured by how much the pupils dilate when observing a scene. When something important appears in one's environment, such as someone with a gun or the person one plans to marry, the pupils dilate, taking in more information. In this study, American military cadets were shown a photo of a potential enemy. For those doing TM, after six months their pupils were more wide open than the controls. This indicates that the TM practice increased their ability to take in more information.

This study also found that six months of TM decreased hypervigilance, which suggests that the increased arousal is appropriate to the situation but not excessive. TM also increased attention to changes that are relevant, and decreased attention to irrelevant factors, both of which are also important for increasing SA.

References: Bandy, C.L., Fleming, K.K., & Dulmage, J. (2013). *Meditation training in rook cadets increases resilience.* Paper presented at the 25th Annual Conference of the Association for Psychological Science, May 23–26 Washington, DC.

Holt, W.R., Caruso, J.L., & Riley, J.B. (1978). Transcendental Meditation vs. pseudo-meditation on visual choice reaction time. *Perceptual and Motor Skills,* 46, 726.

Batorski, M. (2011). Developing situation awareness capacity to improve judgment and decision-making under stress. (Published doctoral dissertation). Pepperdine University. Malibu, CA.

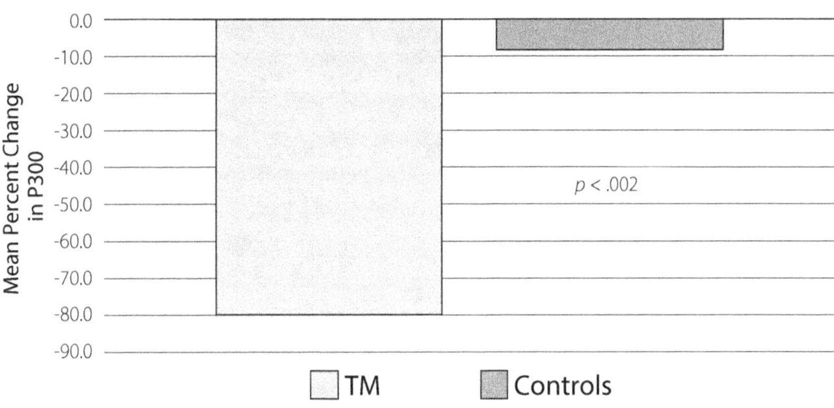

tm-020

IMPROVED FOCUS ON THE IMPORTANT THINGS

Situation awareness (SA) means accurately perceiving what is going on around you, making sense of it in real-time, and then rapidly projecting what will happen next. For example, when juggling plates, you need to be aware of the plates (perception), where they are in relation to each other (comprehension), and where your hands need to be at each moment (projection). If your perception is overwhelmed, or your assessment of where plates are in relation to one another becomes inaccurate, or you momentarily become distracted, your hands will not be where they need to be and you will drop the plates.

The P300 is a brain potential that typically indicates recognition. During an auditory task designed to measure attention without distraction, after six months of TM practice the TM group showed accurate attention with 80% less distraction than the control group. This shows that regular experience of the holistic changes produced by TM practice improves the ability to avoid distraction.

The same study also showed that TM increased awareness of relevant stimuli. (Reference 1) Related studies have shown that TM practice increases field independence, the ability to remain focused on the target and not get distracted by other information coming from the environment.

Other research on SA, looking at perception (ability to appreciate more from one's surroundings), comprehension (making sense of problems faster), and projection (sensing solutions more rapidly), found that after three months of TM, cadets showed statistically significant improvements in perception and projection. (Reference 2)

Reference 1: Bandy, C.L., Fleming, K.K., & Dulmage, J. (2013). *Meditation training in rook cadets increases resilience.* Paper presented at the 25th Annual Conference of the Association for Psychological Science, May 23–26 Washington, DC.

Reference 2: Batorski, M. (2011). Developing situation awareness capacity to improve judgment and decision-making under stress. (Published doctoral dissertation). Pepperdine University. Malibu, CA.

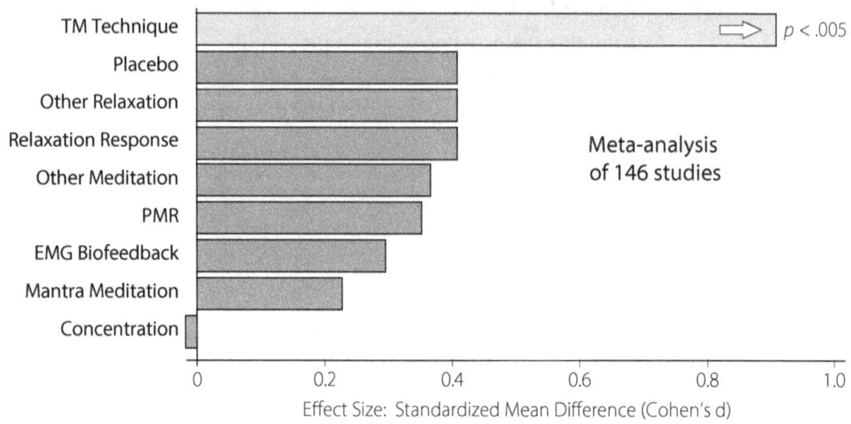

LESS ANXIETY & WORRY

Trait anxiety refers to how anxious a person usually is. A major review done at Stanford University (a meta-analysis of 146 studies), published in the *Journal of Clinical Psychology*, found that the Transcendental Meditation (TM) technique is the most effective technique known for reducing trait anxiety. It is more than twice as effective as all other meditation and relaxation techniques, including Progressive Relaxation, Concentration Meditation, the Relaxation Response (Benson's technique), EMG Biofeedback, and placebo techniques.

A placebo technique is a sham treatment, such as a sugar pill, which has no active ingredient. However, expectations of good results from placebos do have healing effects, as seen in this study. Placebos illustrate the power of mind over matter and doctors recognize how important it is to give the patient hope and to encourage them to be positive, because it helps the healing process. TM was the only technique that produced a stronger effect than the placebo techniques. This is because TM produces a wide range of specific physiological changes which, taken together, are the opposite of the stress response. (Reference 1)

Similarly, more recent meta-analyses have found that TM produces stronger reductions in trait anxiety than mindfulness meditations and other meditations. (Reference 2)

Reference 1: Eppley, K., Abrams A.I., Shear J. Differential effects of relaxation techniques on trait anxiety: A meta-analysis. *Journal of Clinical Psychology* 45, no. 6 (1989): 957–974.

Reference 2: Sedlmeier, P., Eberth, J., Schwarz, M., Zimmermann, D., & Haarig, F. (2012). The psychological effects of meditation: A meta-analysis. *Psychological Bulletin* 138, no. 6 (2012): 1139–1171.

Orme-Johnson, D.W., & Barnes, V.A. Effects of the Transcendental Meditation technique on trait anxiety: A meta-analysis of randomized controlled trials. *Journal of Alternative and Complementary Medicine*, 20, no. 5, (2013): 330–341.

Improved Interaction with the Environment

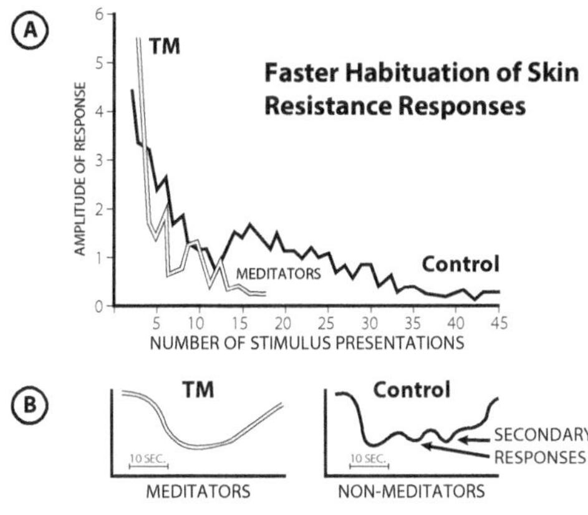

Skin Resistance Response to Stressful Stimuli
(100 dB, 3000 Hz, .5 sec.)

FASTER RECOVERY FROM STRESS

Subjects who practiced the Transcendental Meditation (TM) technique were compared to non-meditating controls of similar age and demographics on how their autonomic nervous systems responded to a series of loud stressful tones. The loud tones were presented while the subjects were sitting quietly with eyes open (not meditating). The stress reaction to each tone was measured by the size (amplitude) of the skin resistance response, which is an aspect of the fight-or-flight startle response, which is measured by sweat on the palms of the hands.

The upper part of the chart (A) shows that the amplitude of the response to the loud tone gets smaller with repeated presentations of it, initially in a similar way for both groups. But then after about the 15th tone, the control group began showing a large startle response again. This is probably because their higher internal stress levels, as indicated by more spontaneous skin resistance responses, was intensifying how they interacted with the environment. In contrast, the TM group was more responsive to the tone when they first heard it, but quite quickly became habituated to it.

The lower part of the chart (B) shows the wave form of the skin resistance response to the first loud tone. It can be seen that the TM group showed a much simpler response than the control group, which showed multiple secondary responses to the loud tone. This illustrates how the internal spontaneous stress responses of the control subjects were worsening how they responded to stress from the environment.

The conclusion is that TM is a way to reduce one's internal stress in order to improve how one experiences stress coming from the environment.

Reference: Orme-Johnson, D.W. (1973). Autonomic stability and Transcendental Meditation. *Psychosomatic Medicine*, 35, 341–349.

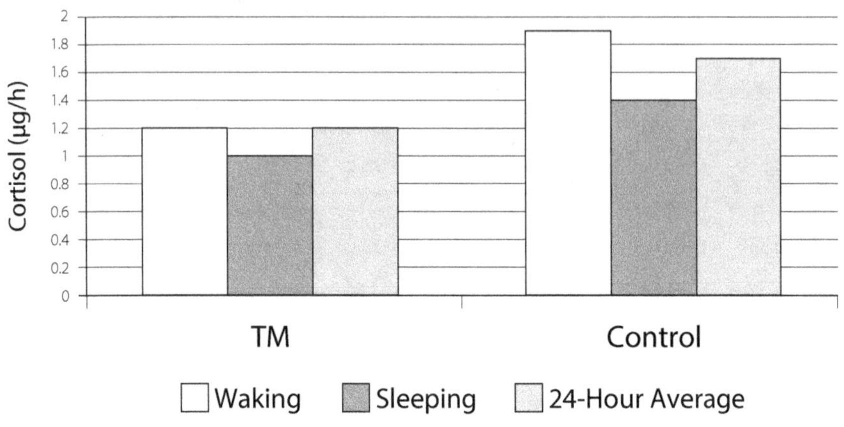

LESS STRESS DAY & NIGHT

Cortisol is the major stress hormone and is an indication of stress during the day. Long-term practitioners of the Transcendental Meditation (TM) technique have lower cortisol levels than non-meditating control subjects throughout the 24-hour cycle of waking and sleeping. The chart above shows that the TM group (left) had lower levels of cortisol than controls (right). (Reference 1)

Lower cortisol may help explain why TM reduces insomnia. As we have seen previously, TM has been shown to reduce insomnia in a number of populations:

- improved sleep quality in executives and workers (Reference 2)

- reduced insomnia in industrial workers (Reference 3)

- improved sleep quality in veterans with PTSD (Reference 4)

- improved sleep quality in prison inmates (Reference 5)

- improved sleep quality in psychiatric patients (Reference 6)

Reference 1: *Journal of Alternative Complementary Medicine,* 1995 1(3):263–83.

Reference 2: *Anxiety, Stress and Coping: An International Journal.* 1993;6:245–62.

Reference 3: *Japanese Journal of Public Health.* 1990;37(10 Suppl.):729.

Reference 4: *Journal of Counseling and Development.* 1985;64:212–5.

Reference 5: *The Permanente Journal.* 2016;20(4):16-007.

Criminal Justice and Behavior. 1978;5:3–20.

Reference 6: *Comparative Psychiatry.* 1975;16(4):303–21.

Reduced Symptoms of Post-Traumatic Stress Disorder

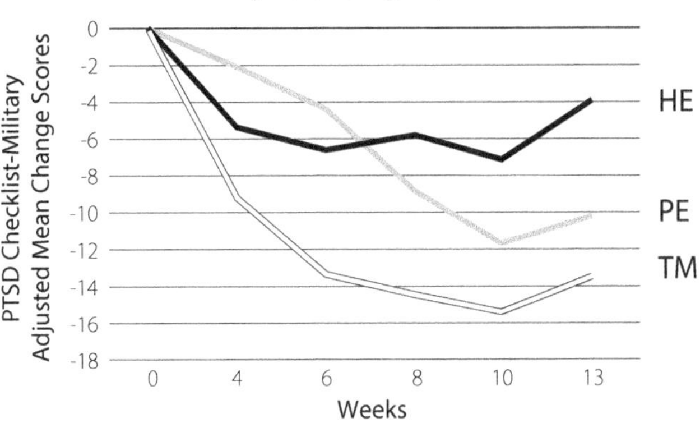

tm-024

RECOVERY FROM TRAUMATIC STRESS

After people have experienced extreme trauma, such as being in a war, they may continue to have serious psychological and physical symptoms, such as flashbacks (vivid feelings that the trauma is happening right now), nightmares about it, intrusive thoughts about it that keep pushing into their minds, and physical sensations such as pain, sweating, nausea, or trembling. These symptoms are collectively known as post-traumatic stress disorder (PTSD). A person with PTSD may even fear that their own shadow is someone trying to attack them. It is a serious and disabling condition that is seen throughout the world, affecting not only war veterans, but also refugees, victims of family violence, prison inmates, minority groups living in racist societies, and many others. PTSD takes a severe toll on the mental, physical, and financial wellbeing of the victims, which is shared by their families.

The Department of Defense office of US Army Medical Research sponsored a $2.4 million study that compared the Transcendental Meditation (TM) technique with Health Education (HE) and the gold standard treatment currently in use by the military, Prolonged Exposure therapy (PE). TM acted more quickly than PE and HE and resulted in more clinically meaningful improvements. Similarly, TM reduced depression more than the comparison techniques. The study was published in one of the world's leading medical journals, *The Lancet Psychiatry*.

A number of other studies also found that TM is highly effective in treating PTSD for war veterans, war refugees, male and female prison inmates, and traumatized college students.

Reference: Nidich, S., Mills, P.J., Rainforth, M., Heppner, P., Schneider, R.H., Rosenthal, N.E., ..., Rutledge, T. (2018). Non-trauma-focused meditation versus exposure therapy in veterans with post-traumatic stress disorder: a randomized controlled trial. *The Lancet Psychiatry*, 5(12), 975–986.

Improved Sleep Quality

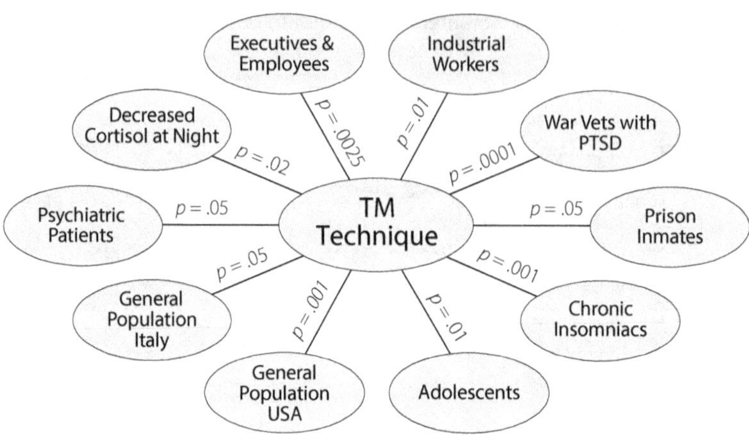

tm-025

SLEEP BETTER, WAKE REFRESHED

Nearly 30% of Americans complain about insomnia. Insomnia causes unclear thinking, poor motor performance, and impaired quality of life. Poor sleep increases healthcare utilization, absenteeism, and accidents, and it presents a substantial financial burden on society. Decades of research have linked chronic sleep deprivation to increased risk for obesity, heart disease, type 2 diabetes, and problems with immune function.

Scientific research indicates that the Transcendental Meditation (TM) technique reduces insomnia by approximately 30%–65% in many populations: business executives and employees, industrial workers, war veterans suffering from PTSD, prison inmates, chronic insomniacs, adolescents, the general population, and psychiatric patients. TM decreases nighttime cortisol, one of the biomedical hallmarks of insomnia, by 40%.

References:

1. *Anxiety, Stress and Coping: An International Journal.* 1993;6:245–62.

2. *Japanese Journal of Public Health.* 1990;37(10 Suppl.):729.

3. *Journal of Counseling and Development.* 1985;64:212–5.

4. *Criminal Justice and Behavior.* 1978;5:3–20.

5. *Scientific Research on the Transcendental Meditation Program: Collected papers*, Vol 1. 1977; paper 41.

6. *Scientific research on Maharishi's Transcendental Meditation and TM-Sidhi Program: Collected papers*, Vol 2. 1978/1989; paper 153.

7. *Scientific Research on Maharishi's Transcendental Meditation and TM-Sidhi Program: Collected papers*, Vol 2. 1976/1989; paper 126.

8. *Scientific research on Maharishi's Transcendental Meditation and TM-Sidhi Program: Collected papers*, Vol 3. 1981; paper 239.

9. *Comparative Psychiatry.* 1975;16(4):303–21.

10. *Journal of Alternative Complementary Medicine.* 1995;1(3):263–83.

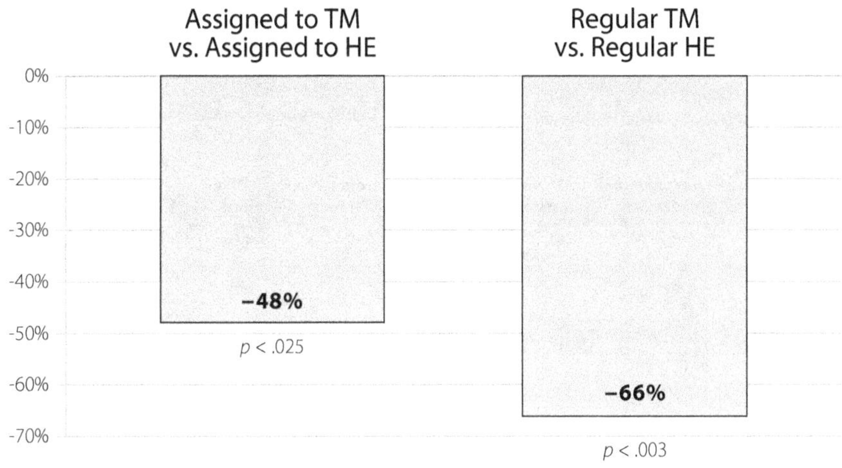

LIVE LONGER, BE HEALTHIER

A study of 201 heart patients found that during an average 5.4-year follow-up, the risk of heart attacks, strokes, and deaths decreased by 48% (p = .025) in the patients who were randomly assigned to the Transcendental Meditation (TM) program, compared to the control subjects randomized to receive health-education classes instead of TM (left bar). On average, both the TM group and the HE groups practiced either TM or healthy life-style activities, respectively, about 8.5 times per week, which is 61% of the recommended twice-a-day practice for both programs.

A high-adherence subgroup analysis was conducted on all 141 patients practicing TM or HE activities once a day or more. The high-adherence TM group had 66% fewer heart attacks, strokes, and deaths in the follow-up period than the high-adherence HE group (p=.003) (right bar).

The study also found a significant inverse correlation between regularity of TM home practice and reduction in heart attacks, strokes, and deaths (p = .04). This means that the more regularly a patient practiced TM, the greater the reduction of risk for future cardiac events.

The TM group also showed a 24% risk reduction compared to the HE group in a composite measure of secondary end points, which included cardiovascular mortality, revascularizations, and cardiovascular hospitalizations; blood pressure; psychosocial stress factors; and lifestyle behaviors (p = 0.17). Compared to the HE group, the TM groups had reductions of 4.9 mm Hg in systolic blood pressure (p = 0.01) and anger expression (p < 0.05 for all scales). Adherence with TM was associated with greater survival.

Reference: Schneider, R.H., Grim, C.E., Rainforth, M.A., et al. "Stress reduction in the secondary prevention of cardiovascular disease: Randomized controlled trial of Transcendental Meditation and health education in Blacks." *Circulation: Cardiovascular Quality Outcomes*, 5, no. 6 (2012): 750–758.

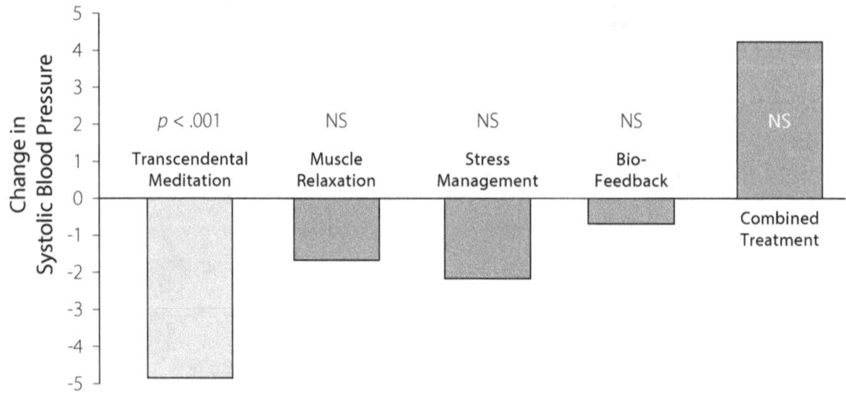

HEALTHIER BLOOD PRESSURE

Reducing stress reduces stress-related disease, including high blood pressure, a major risk factor for heart disease, which is the world's No. 1 killer. According to research, high blood pressure is almost entirely preventable. This comprehensive meta-analysis of published, high-quality randomized controlled trials found that the Transcendental Meditation (TM) technique was the only stress-reduction program that significantly reduced blood pressure in hypertensive patients.

The American Heart Association (AHA) scientific review of alternative treatments for high blood pressure concluded that TM is recommended for consideration in treatment plans for all individuals with blood pressure > 120/80 mm Hg. The AHA scientific statement also reported the finding that lower blood pressure through TM practice is associated with substantially reduced rates of death, heart attack, and stroke.

In 2013, the American Heart Association said "...The evidence to date supports using TM practice to help reduce high blood pressure. Other meditations do not show as strong an effect on reducing hypertension.... The Transcendental Meditation technique is the only meditation practice that has been shown to lower blood pressure ... all other meditation techniques (including MBSR*) ... are not recommended in clinical practice to lower blood pressure at this time."

*MBSR refers to Mindfulness Based Stress Reduction, the most widely used mindfulness technique in clinical settings.

References: Rainforth, M.V., Schneider, R.H., Nidich, S.I., Gaylord-King, C., Salerno, J.W., Anderson, J.W. Stress reduction programs in patients with elevated blood pressure: A systematic review and meta-analysis. *Current Hypertension Reports.* 2007;9(6):520–8.

Brook, R.D. et al., Beyond Medications and Diet: Alternative Approaches to Lowering Blood Pressure. A Scientific Statement from the American Heart Association. *Hypertension*, 61:00, 2013.

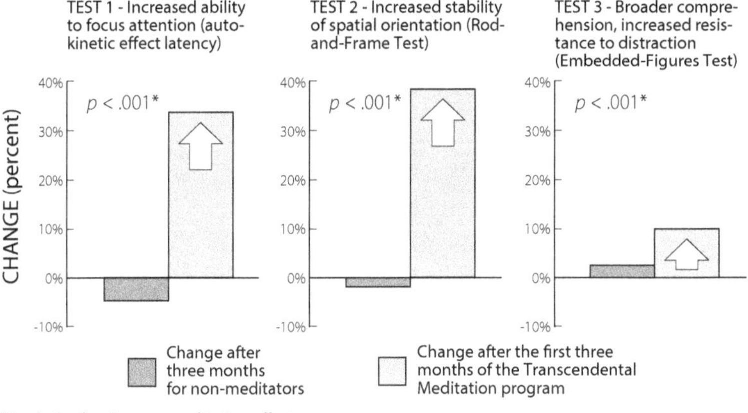

BROADER COMPREHENSION & IMPROVED ABILITY TO FOCUS ATTENTION

In this study three tests were administered that directly measure field independence, the ability to focus attention on specific objects without being distracted by the environment of the objects. Subjects changed significantly in the direction of increased field independence after practicing the Transcendental Meditation (TM) technique for three months, compared with a non-meditating control group.

The latency of the autokinetic effect measures the time it takes a subject to perceive movement of a spot of light (Test 1 in the chart above); the Rod-and-Frame Test measures the ability to orient a rod to true vertical position against a tilted frame (Test 2); and the Embedded-Figures Test measures the ability to perceive simple figures embedded in a complex background (Test 3).

These measures indicate the development of field independence, the ability to analytically perceive an item embedded in a complex context. Researchers have found that persons with greater field independence have the following characteristics: greater ability to assimilate and structure experience; greater organization of mind and cognitive clarity; improved memory; greater creative expression; stable internal frame of reference; stable standards, attitudes, judgment, and sentiments without continuous reference to external standards; differentiation of inner and outer; autonomic stability; more assertiveness. All these characteristics are indications of improved neurological organization and, consequently, more evolved consciousness. This improvement in TMers is all the more remarkable because it was previously believed that these basic perceptual abilities do not improve beyond early adulthood.

References: Pelletier, K.R., "The Effects of the Transcendental Meditation Program on Perceptual Style: Increased Field Independence," In Orme-Johnson, D.W. & Farrow, J.T. (Eds.), *Scientific Research on the Transcendental Meditation Program: Collected papers* (Vol. 1, pp. 337–345). Maharishi European Research University Press (1977).

Pelletier, K.R., "Influence of Transcendental Meditation upon Autokinetic Perception," *Perceptual and Motor Skills* 39 (1974): 1031–1034.

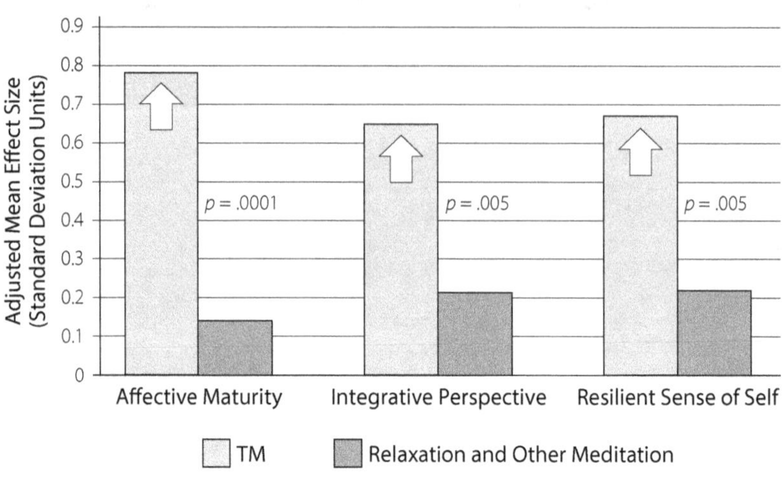

tm-029

BE MORE SELF-SUFFICIENT

Affective (emotional) maturity denotes a person capable of engaging in appropriate, balanced, responsible, and productive relationships with other people, in a wide variety of situations.

Integrative perspective portrays an individual who has a positive view of self and humanity, who can integrate dichotomies, and who embraces higher values such as the good in oneself and others.

Resilient sense of self indicates an individual who maintains a stable internal frame of reference, whose awareness is in the "here and now," and who responds adaptively to both internal and external challenges.

Self-actualized people respond based on who they know they are, rather than on changing their behavior to fit in. They bring their best thinking to all their behavior.

The deep rest of TM removes stress and fatigue and allows the individual to grow toward their full human potential, displaying all these components of self-actualization.

With daily practice of TM, people come to feel good about themselves and recognize that people everywhere in the world are also good. They come to experience that the inner self in everyone is an unbounded ocean of happiness and creative intelligence, even though people differ in skin color, language, food, behavior, customs, and religious beliefs. They come to understand that everyone else is also growing at their own pace, and will ultimately express their inner Self as happiness and love. For the enlightened, *the world is their family*.

Reference: Alexander, C.N., Rainforth, M.V., & Gelderloos, P. (1991). Transcendental Meditation, Self-Actualization and Psychological Health: A Conceptual Overview and Statistical Meta-Analysis, *Journal of Social Behavior and Personality* 6(5), 189–247.

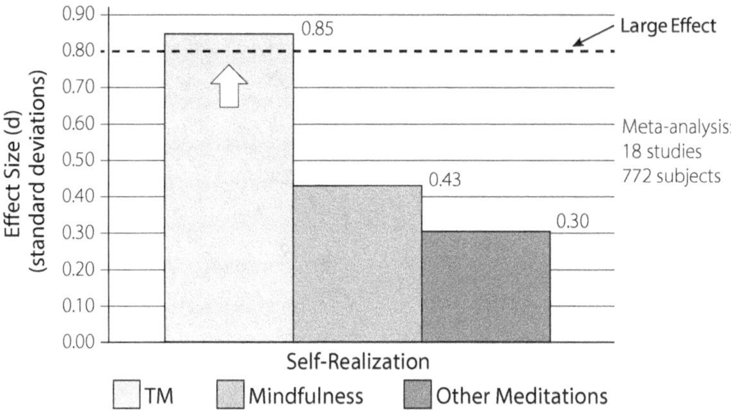

BE MORE YOURSELF

Self-realization (understood as self-actualization) refers to realizing one's full inner potential, expressed in every area of life. A well-controlled statistical meta-analysis of 18 studies on 722 subjects indicated that the effect of the Transcendental Meditation (TM) program on increasing self-realization is significantly greater than mindfulness or other forms of meditation. (Reference 1) This study replicates the findings of an earlier exhaustive meta-analysis (42 studies), which also found that TM has a large effect approximately three times that of other forms of meditation and relaxation. This study also found that TM produced greater effects than other meditation and relaxation techniques, with substantial increases in self-actualization in just three months. (Reference 2)

TM has been shown to increase self-actualization in populations ranging from administrators in the USA (Reference 3) to disadvantaged women in Uganda (Reference 4). The study in Uganda found that after 3 months the women practicing the TM technique showed decreased perceived stress and increased self-efficacy compared to a control group who waited until after the study to learn TM.

Brain research has found that the psychological changes produced by TM practice are associated with increased connectivity of relevant brain areas. (Reference 5) These studies suggest that the increase in self-actualization through TM practice is based on a re-wiring of the brain to function in a more stress-free, integrated, holistic fashion—a new brain for a new life.

Reference 1: *Psychological Bulletin*, 2012 138(6), 1139–1171.

Reference 2: *Journal of Social Behavior and Personality*, 1991 6(5), 189–247.

Reference 3: *The Permanente Journal*, 2018 E-pub: 10/29/2018.

Reference 4: *Health Care Women International*, 2018 March 1:1–24.

Reference 5: *Brain and Cognition*, Vol. 139 2020 March 139, 1–11.

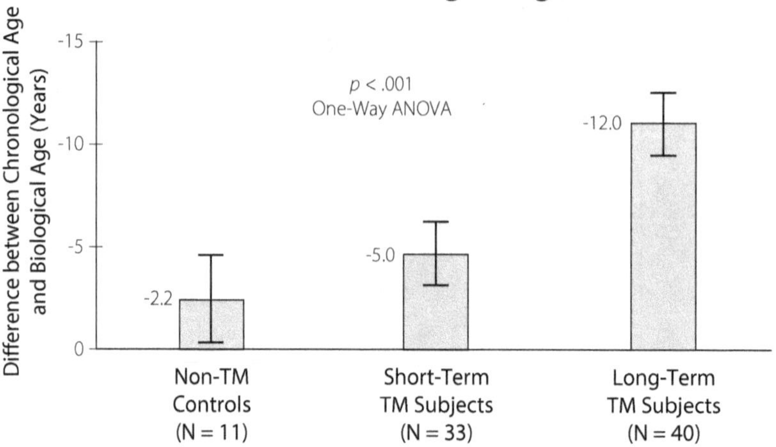

tm-031

SLOWING DOWN THE AGING PROCESS

A standardized test of biological age, the Adult Growth Examination, was given to a cross-sectional group of men and women with a mean age of 53 years. They were divided into three groups: non-meditating controls, short-term TMers (under five years) and long-term TMers (over five years). The average biological age of the non-meditating controls was 2.6 years younger than their chronological age; of the short-term TMers, 5.0 years younger than their chronological age; of the long-term TMers, 12.0 years younger.

A statistically significant difference was found between the long-term TMers and both the control group and short-term TMers (F = 8.05, p<.001, one-way ANOVA). Further, a significant correlation (r = .46, p<.001) was found between younger biological age and length of time practicing the TM technique.

These findings suggest that practice of the TM technique slows or reverses the aging process—and that the longer one practices the TM technique, the younger one's biological age when compared with chronological age. The deep rest experienced during the TM technique allows the physiology to dissolve stress. As a result, mind and body become more stable, adaptable, and integrated—less susceptible to wear and tear—and the aging process is reduced and reversed.

Reference: Wallace, R.K., Jacobe, E., & Harrington, B. The Effects of the Transcendental Meditation and TM-Sidhi Program on the Aging Process. *International Journal of Neuroscience*, 16 (1) 1982: 53-58.

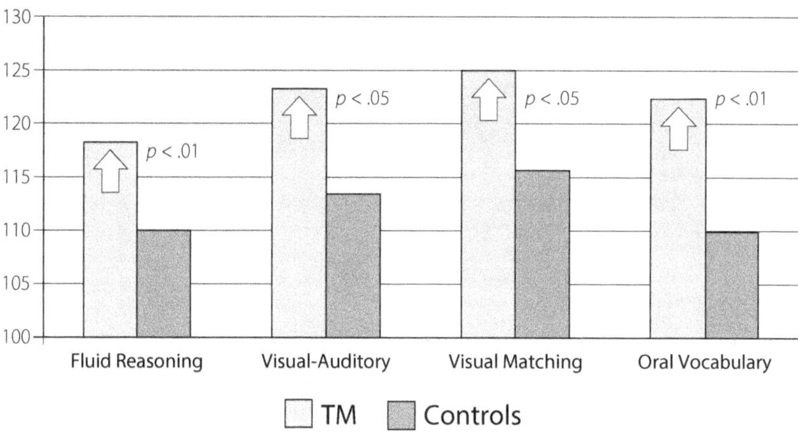

tm-032

CLEARER MIND WITH INCREASING AGE

It is a common experience that there is usually a decline in cognitive functioning in the elderly. This study of elders between the ages of 60 and 74, however, found that those practicing the Transcendental Meditation (TM) program exhibited significantly higher levels of fluid reasoning, verbal intelligence, long-term memory, and speed of processing than matched controls.

Further analyses found that the TM group had lower levels of the free radical lipid peroxide. Lipid peroxide is composed of highly reactive oxygen-rich molecules, called free radicals, which "steal" electrons from important compounds (fatty acids/lipids) in cell membranes, resulting in cell damage. The chemical products of this oxidation are known as lipid peroxides or lipid oxidation products. This process plays a major part in the development of chronic and degenerative conditions such as cancer, autoimmune disorders, aging, cataracts, rheumatoid arthritis, and cardiovascular and neurodegenerative diseases.

The study also showed significant correlations with lipid peroxide levels for both reasoning ability and memory, suggesting a possible link between cognitive functioning and free radical activity in the elderly. The study also illustrates that TM produces holistic changes ranging from basic biochemical mechanisms underlying health to the highest levels of brain integration that underlie human perception and reasoning.

Reference: Nidich, S.I., Schneider, R.H., Nidich, R.J., Foster, G., Sharma, H., Salerno, J.W., ..., Alexander, C.N. (2005). Effect of the Transcendental Meditation program on intellectual development in community-dwelling older adults. *Journal of Social Behavior and Personality*, 17(1), 217–228.

Reversal of Aging

through the Transcendental Meditation program

PHYSIOLOGY	Through aging	Through TM
Blood pressure	↗	↘
Auditory threshold	↗	↘
Near-point vision	↗	↘
Cardiovascular efficiency	↘	↗
Cerebral blood flow	↘	↗
Homeostatic recovery	↘	↗

BIOCHEMISTRY		
Cholesterol concentration	↗	↘
Hemoglobin concentration	↘	↗

MIND-BODY COORDINATION		
Reaction time	↗	↘
Sensory-motor performance	↘	↗

Reversal of Aging

through the Transcendental Meditation program

PSYCHOLOGY	Through aging	Through TM
Susceptibility to stress	↗	↘
Behavioral rigidity	↗	↘
Learning ability	↘	↗
Memory	↘	↗
Creativity	↘	↗
Intelligence	↘	↗

HEALTH		
Cardiovascular disease	↗	↘
Hypertension	↗	↘
Asthma (severity)	↗	↘
Insomnia	↗	↘
Depression	↗	↘
Immune system efficiency	↘	↗
Quality of sleep	↘	↗

All these factors show deterioration with the aging process. The opposite changes — indicating a reversal of the aging process — are observed with the Transcendental Meditation program.

LONGEVITY FACTOR → **CARDIO-VASCULAR HEALTH** · **WORK SATIS-FACTION** · **POSITIVE HEALTH HABITS**

IMPROVEMENTS OCCURRING AS A RESULT OF THE TRANSCENDENTAL MEDITATION AND TM-SIDHI PROGRAM	CARDIO-VASCULAR HEALTH	WORK SATIS-FACTION	POSITIVE HEALTH HABITS
	Decreased hypertension	Increased job satisfaction	Decreased cigarette smoking
	Improvements in patients with angina pectoris	Improved relationships with supervisors and peers	Decreased alcohol consumption
	Decreased cholesterol level	Improved job performance	Decreased use of non-prescribed drugs
	Increased cardiovascular efficiency	Increased ego strength	
		Increased self-esteem	
		Increased self-reliance	

The eight factors shown above have been found to be most clearly showing improvements related to longevity. The research results listed beneath each factor, in all these areas, indicate the stabilization of perfect health and the promotion of longevity through the Transcendental Meditation and TM-Sidhi program.

# of Longevity

TM program

<table>
<tr><td>PHYSICAL FUNCTION</td><td>HAPPINESS RATING</td><td>SELF HEALTH RATING</td><td>INTELLIGENCE</td><td>MENTAL HEALTH</td></tr>
<tr><td>Improved auditory thresholds</td><td>Increased happiness</td><td>Improvements in self health rating (in addition to improvements in objective measurements of health)</td><td>Increased intelligence</td><td>Improvements in psychological health</td></tr>
<tr><td>Enhanced perceptual ability</td><td>Increased contentment</td><td></td><td>Increased creativity</td><td>Decreased anxiety</td></tr>
<tr><td>Faster reaction time</td><td>Increased self-regard</td><td></td><td></td><td>Decreased neuroticism and depression</td></tr>
<tr><td>Improvements in patients with bronchial asthma</td><td>Increased adaptability to life events</td><td></td><td></td><td></td></tr>
<tr><td>Increased vital capacity</td><td></td><td></td><td></td><td></td></tr>
<tr><td>Improved running speed and agility</td><td></td><td></td><td></td><td></td></tr>
<tr><td>Improved perceptual-motor performance</td><td></td><td></td><td></td><td></td></tr>
<tr><td>Reduced inflammation</td><td></td><td></td><td></td><td></td></tr>
<tr><td>Relief from insomnia</td><td></td><td></td><td></td><td></td></tr>
<tr><td>Faster recovery from stress</td><td></td><td></td><td></td><td></td></tr>
<tr><td>Improved biochemical stability, homeostasis, & efficiency</td><td></td><td></td><td></td><td></td></tr>
<tr><td>Restful style of physiological functioning</td><td></td><td></td><td></td><td></td></tr>
</table>

The first seven factors shown above in order of importance were identified by a major study (E. Palmore, 1974, *Normal Aging II*, Durham: Duke University Press. USA.) to be closely related to longevity. The last factor, mental health, has been found to be of great importance for longevity and good health in later life (Valliant, G.E., *New England Journal of Medicine*, 1979, 301,1249–1254).

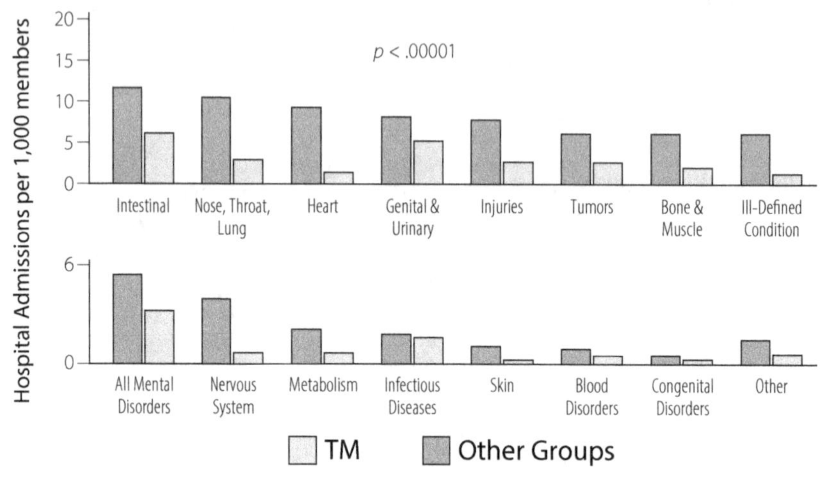

LESS NEED FOR HEALTH CARE

This study compared five years of health statistics of 2,000 people practicing the Transcendental Meditation (TM) program compared to normative data, which is the average of all 600,000 people covered by the insurance company. The chart above compares the hospitalization rate of the TM group (light bars) with the normative data (dark bars). It can be seen in the chart that the TM group had lower hospitalization rates in all categories of disease, by an average of approximately 50% overall. Reductions in the TM group included 87% less hospitalization for heart disease, 55% less for cancer, 87% less for diseases of the nervous system, and 65% less for metabolic disease. Similar results were found comparing the TM group with a control group matched for age and profession, indicating that the results for TM were not due to age or type of profession.

The results for outpatient medical care utilization (doctor visits) and medical costs were similar to the results for hospitalization, approximately 50% lower for the TM group than the norm.

The subjects in this study had been doing TM for about 5 years, which suggests that their medical utilization and costs were decreasing at a rate of about 10% per year over the 5-year period in the TM group. (Reference 1) This was confirmed by a 14-year study of 1,418 people before and after they learned TM compared to 1,418 matched non-meditating controls. In the eight years before the TM group learned TM, their medical care costs were not different from the control group. However, after they learned TM, their medical care costs decreased by an average of 14% per year relative to controls. (Reference 2)

Reference 1: Orme-Johnson, D.W. (1987). Medical care utilization and the Transcendental Meditation program. *Psychosomatic Medicine*, 49, 493–507.

Reference 2: Herron, R., & Hillis, S. (2000). The impact of the Transcendental Meditation program on government payments to physicians in Quebec: An update. *American Journal of Health Promotion*, 14(5), 284–293.

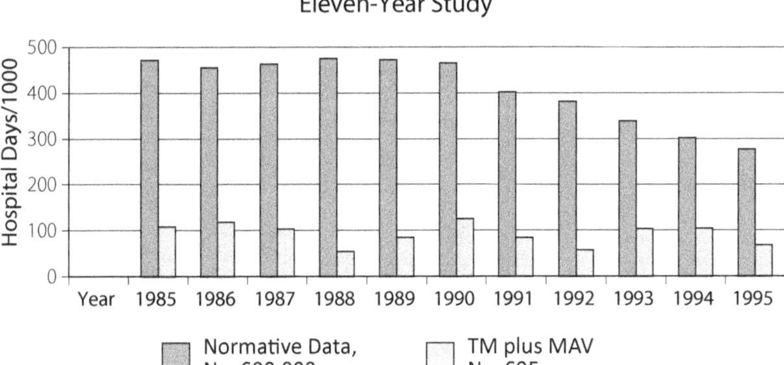

MUCH LESS NEED TO BE IN THE HOSPITAL

This was an eleven-year study of health insurance statistics* on a group of 695 people practicing the Transcendental Meditation (TM) program plus other modalities of Maharishi AyurVeda (MAV), such as yoga exercises, herbal massage, and dietary recommendations. The TM plus MAV group was compared to the normative database of the insurance company. The study found that the rate of hospitalization by all causes for the TM plus MAV group was consistently much lower than the norm year after year, on average 74% lower. (Reference 1) The study also found that outpatient care for the TM plus MAV group was also consistently lower than for the norm over the eleven years, on average 55% lower.

The same study also found that medical expenditures were consistently lower than the norm over the years, by 62%.

Health care costs increase with age. TM practice reduces costs in this group. A study of medical expenditures for people over 65 found that after learning TM, the TMers' medical costs decreased 14% per year, to 70% less than controls after only five years. (Reference 2)

These studies show that any nation would save billions of dollars if the TM program were made available as a tool for stress reduction to everyone.

Reference 1: Orme-Johnson, D.W., & Herron, R.E. (1997). An innovative approach to reducing medical care utilization and expenditures. *The American Journal of Managed Care*, 3(1), 135–144.

***Note:** Data courtesy of Blue Cross Blue Shield of Iowa.

Reference 2: Herron, R.E., & Cavanaugh, K. (2005). Can the Transcendental Meditation program reduce the medical expenditures of older people? A longitudinal cost reduction study in Canada. *Journal of Social Behavior and Personality*, 17, 415–442.

Reduced Medical Utilization in All Age Categories

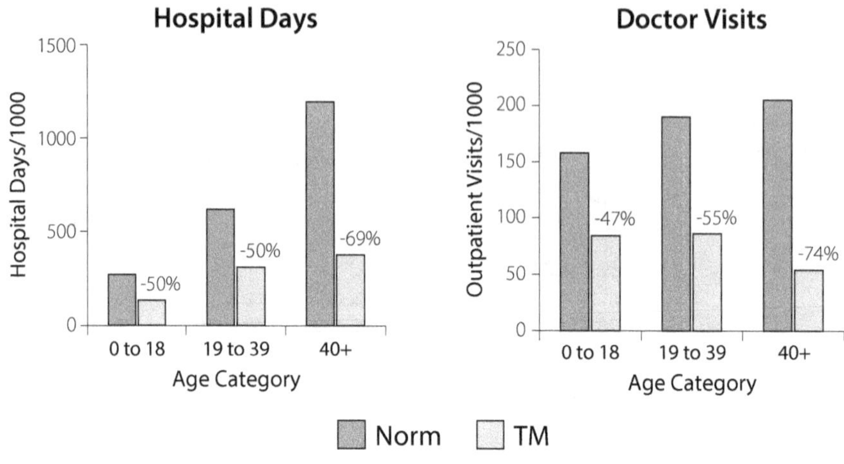

BETTER HEALTH ACROSS THE LIFESPAN

Better health for all age groups. The data from a health insurance company* showed that a group of 2,000 people practicing the Transcendental Meditation (TM) technique had fewer days in the hospital and fewer doctor visits in all age categories. This indicates that the lower rates of sickness for the TM group were not because the TM group was younger. It also shows that TM is an effective tool for helping prevent diseases for people of all ages. Interestingly, the largest decreases were for the oldest group: 69% fewer days spent in the hospital and 74% fewer doctor visits. By comparison to normative data, TM-group children (0–18 years old) and TM-group young adults had about a 50% reduction in hospitalization and doctor visits compared to non-meditating people of their age. (Reference 1)

A number of other studies have also indicated that practicing TM slows biological aging.

Younger biological age. A landmark study provided evidence that TM decreases biological age. The study found that a group that had been doing TM an average of 3 years had a biological age 5 years younger than their chronological age. A group doing TM for 7 years had a biological age 12 years younger. (Reference 2)

Decreased mortality. TM reduces the death rate, also called the mortality rate. One eight-year study found that the TM group had 19% fewer deaths than control groups. (Reference 3) A second study followed up older blood pressure patients a maximum of 18.8 years and found that the TM group showed a 23% decrease in deaths by all causes. (Reference 4)

Reference 1: *Psychosomatic Medicine* 1987;49:493–507.

*****Note:** Data courtesy of Blue Cross Blue Shield of Iowa.

Reference 2: *International Journal of Neuroscience.* 16, 53–58.

Reference 3: *Journal of Social Behavior and Personality.* 2005;17(1):201–16.

Reference 4: *American Journal of Cardiology.* 2005;95(9):1060–4.

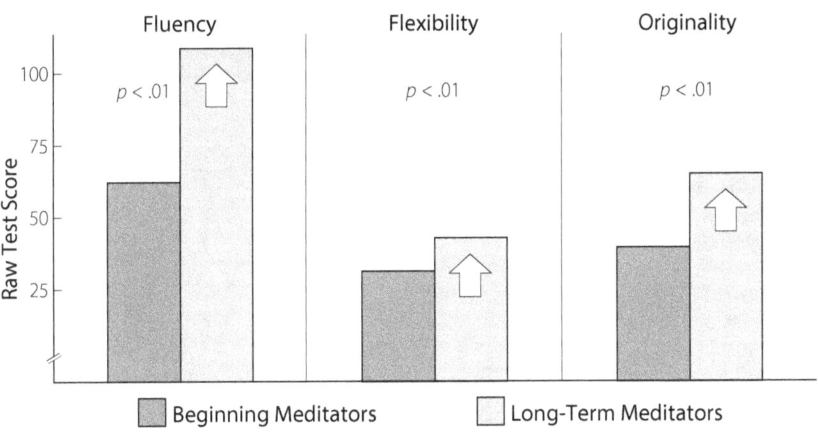

INCREASED CREATIVITY

The Torrance Test of Creative Thinking (TTCT), Verbal Form A, was used to compare 44 subjects practicing the Transcendental Meditation (TM) technique for an average of 18 months with 41 subjects who had just learned TM.

The two groups were equivalent in age, sex, education, and income level. The long-term TMers scored significantly higher (p <.01) on all three scales of the TTCT—Fluency, Flexibility, and Originality—indicating that practice of the Transcendental Meditation technique increases creativity.

The TTCT was developed to measure the type of creative thinking process described by eminent scientific researchers, inventors, and creative writers. Psychologists such as Carl Rogers and Abraham Maslow have associated this type of creativity with increased self-actualization, which has also been found by independent studies to result from the TM program.

These findings give objective validation to the statement that TM systematically develops creative intelligence by providing a means to directly experience the source of creativity in the mind. The aspects of creativity measured here—fluency, flexibility, and originality—may be associated with integration, adaptability, and growth, three of the fundamentals of progress that are enhanced by TM.

Reference: MacCallum, M.J. (1974/1977). The Transcendental Meditation program and creativity. In Orme-Johnson, D.W. & Farrow, J. (Eds.), *Scientific Research on the Transcendental Meditation Program, Collected papers* (Vol. 1, pp. 410–414). Maharishi European Research University Press (1977).

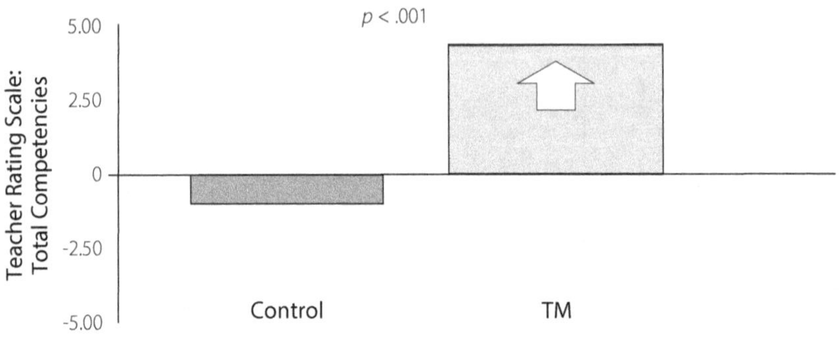

tm-037

BETTER EMOTIONAL & COPING SKILLS

Social-emotional competence is the ability to interact with others, regulate one's own emotions and behavior, solve problems, and communicate effectively. These are skills that it benefits a person to learn early in life in order that all of their relationships are more effective and fulfilling. More successful and fulfilling relationships foster increased self-confidence and self-esteem.

This study found that the Transcendental Meditation (TM) technique accelerated the natural development of social-emotional skills in sixth graders. The study was undertaken because of a growing body of research showing that the widely implemented Quiet Time program, which includes TM, improves positive emotional and behavioral coping skills, resilience, and self-actualization.

Both teacher ratings of social-emotional competencies and student self-reported psychological symptoms of distress and other emotional symptoms improved in the TM group compared to controls after four months of TM practice. (Reference 1)

Other studies on social behavior found:

- **Improved work relations** in executives and workers (Reference 2)

- **Improved behavior** in inner-city children after four months (Reference 3)

- **Decreased dropout rate and increased graduation rate** in inner-city high school students (Reference 4)

- **Decreased hostility** in Folsom maximum-security prisoners (Reference 5)

Reference 1: *Education.* 2019:139(3), 111–119.

Reference 2: *Health Quality Life Outcomes.* 2003:1(1):10.

Reference 3: *Education.* 2013:133(4), 495–501.

Reference 4: 1993: *Anxiety, Stress and Coping: An International Journal.* 6, 245–262.

Reference 5: 1971: *Criminal Justice and Behavior.* 6(1), 13–21.

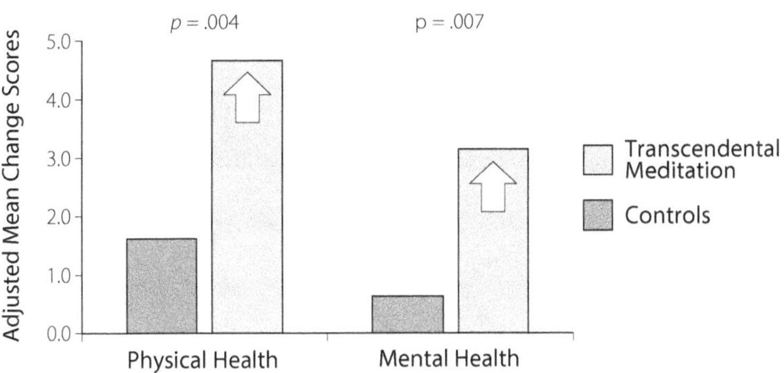

tm-038

BETTER HEALTH, LESS WORRY, MORE HAPPINESS

This study on the effects of the Transcendental Meditation technique on self-efficacy, perceived stress, and quality of life of mothers living in poverty in Uganda was a collaboration between the United Women's Platform and Empowerment and Development (UWOPED), the African Women and Girls Organization for Total Knowledge, Uganda Ltd. (a TM teaching organization in Uganda), and Maharishi International University in Fairfield, Iowa. In this controlled trial, 81 disadvantaged Ugandan women were assigned to TM or a Wait-List Control. The study found that after 3 months the women practicing TM showed increased physical and mental health, as measured by the Medical Outcomes Survey (35 items) using physical and mental health subscales. These changes reflect greater energy and vitality, and greater ability to think clearly, concentrate, plan, and make decisions.

Brenda Nakalembe, Founder and Executive Director of UWOPED said: "Before offering TM we had some success with our programs for the mothers, but had to work hard to inspire and engage them in activities to better themselves, and often they would not continue because of being depressed or unable to function in their lives. Now, with the addition of the TM training I see that mothers are experiencing greater emotional stability, less anger, clearer thinking, happiness, and well-being, and they are more motivated and engaged in taking care of themselves and their children. It is quite remarkable, and they report that their families are more harmonious and that they have less conflict with their neighbors. Seeing changes in their neighbors has brought more and more women to UWOPED to take part in all of our training, especially the TM training."

Reference: Goldstein, L., Nidich, S., Goodman, R., & Goodman, D. H. (2018). The effect of Transcendental Meditation on self-efficacy, perceived stress, and quality of life of mothers in Uganda. *Health Care for Women International, published online: 18 Apr 2018.*

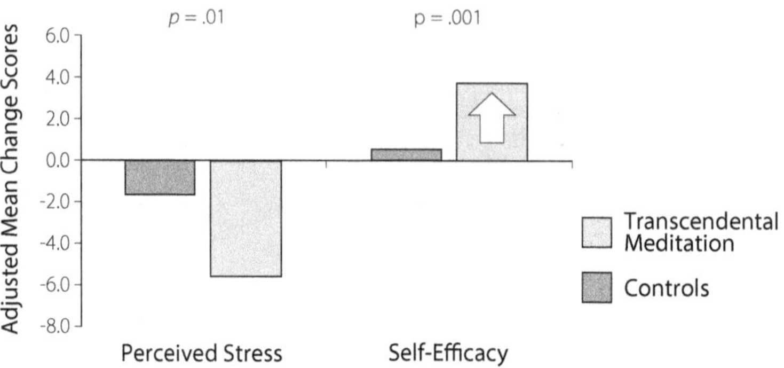

tm-039

MORE EFFECTIVE THOUGHT & ACTION

The same controlled trial with 81 disadvantaged women in Uganda that found improvement in their physical and mental health also found that TM practice decreased their perceived stress and increased their self-efficacy.

"Perceived self-efficacy means if you think you can do something you can do it," explains lead researcher Dr. Leslee Goldstein. "It's really that simple. People with high self-efficacy think they can accomplish tasks. And that's one of the major findings of this study — that self-efficacy was significantly higher after just three months of TM practice."

The rise in measures of self-efficacy was especially marked considering the state of worthlessness, hopelessness and dependence that these women reported before the study. These self-empowered women are taking new directions, finding work, and not feeling dependent on others for their survival.

Dr. Goldstein highlights an important discovery of the study: empowerment has to come from the inside. "You can't empower another person. These women are finding a beautiful source of peace and strength from within themselves just by closing their eyes and practicing the TM technique twice a day. This is giving them the inner strength to persevere, become resilient, and move forward based on their own internal resources."

Reference: Goldstein, L., Nidich, S., Goodman, R., & Goodman, D.H. (2018). The effect of Transcendental Meditation on self-efficacy, perceived stress, and quality of life of mothers in Uganda. *Health Care for Women International, Published online: 18 Apr 2018.*

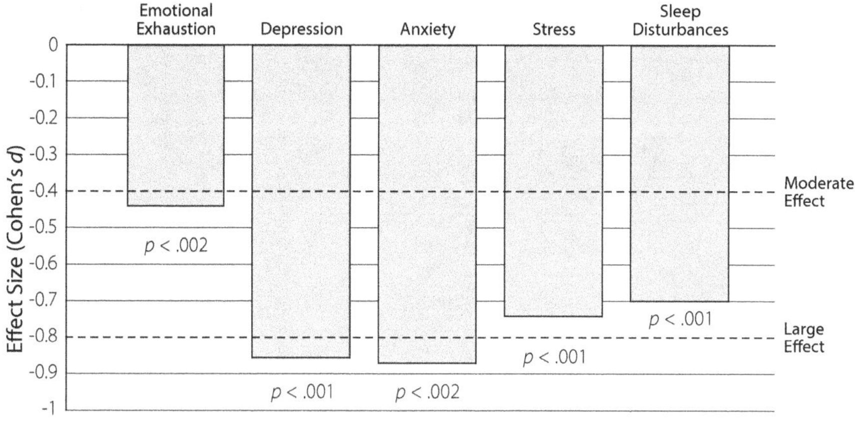

FUNCTION BETTER IN STRESSFUL SITUATIONS

Emergency clinicians face elevated rates of burnout that result in poor outcomes for clinicians, patients, and health systems. During the coronavirus disease 2019 (COVID-19) pandemic, thirty-two emergency clinicians (physicians, nurses, and physician-assistants) from two urban hospitals were recruited to participate in Transcendental Meditation (TM) program for 3 months. Participants demonstrated significant reductions in burnout and in symptoms of emotional exhaustion—decreased depression, anxiety, stress, and sleep disturbance.

93% said TM was helpful during COVID and that they would recommend TM to a friend.

This study replicates previous research indicating that TM practice increases resilience. The way TM increases resilience is that, during TM, stress, as measured by physiological stress markers, is reduced. Further, regular TM develops a calmer style of physiological functioning during activity. It reduces anxiety, accelerates recovery from stress, increases brainwave coherence, and increases creativity, fluid intelligence, and practical intelligence. All these changes contribute to increasing one's resilience.

This study found that TM training was feasible for emergency clinicians during the COVID-19 pandemic and that it led to significant increases in resilience and reductions in burnout and psychological symptoms. TM is a safe and effective meditation tool to provide prolonged improvements in resilience and decreased burnout for clinicians.

Reference: Azizoddin, D.R., Kvaternik, N., Beck, M., Zhou, G., Hasdianda, M.A., Jones, N., Johnsky, L., Im, D., Chai, P.R., & Boyer, E.W. (2021). Heal the Healers: A pilot study evaluating the feasibility, acceptability, and exploratory efficacy of a Transcendental Meditation intervention for emergency clinicians during the coronavirus disease 2019 pandemic. *Journal of the American College of Emergency Physicians Open*, 2(6), e12619.

MORE RESILIENCE UNDER PRESSURE

Researchers based at Sarasota Memorial Hospital in Florida USA collaborated with TM for Nurses to conduct a four-month study of the effects of the Transcendental Meditation (TM) technique on 27 nurses. They found clear statistical evidence that TM increased resilience and "compassion satisfaction," which is the pleasure and satisfying feeling that comes from helping others. The study also demonstrated that TM decreased burnout and secondary traumatic stress, which is the emotional distress that results when an individual hears about the trauma experiences of another. (Reference 1)

A follow-up randomized control trial of 104 nurses in three Florida hospitals showed that, after three months, the TM group demonstrated significantly higher flourishing and mindful awareness, and significantly lower levels of PTSD, anxiety, and burnout. The symptoms of secondary traumatic stress mimic those of post-traumatic stress disorder. (Reference 2)

Previous research has found that TM practice is highly effective in reducing PTSD symptoms in war veterans and refugees, male and female prison inmates, and traumatized college students. These two studies now show the effectiveness of nurses' practice of the TM technique to reduce PTSD, secondary traumatic stress, anxiety, and burnout, and improve compassion, satisfaction, resilience, flourishing, and mindful awareness. TM provides nurses with a simple and effective, evidence-based strategy for enhancing well-being, with the goal of retaining clinical nurses in practice.

Reference 1: Bonamer, J.R., & Aquino-Russell, C. (2019 May/April). Self-care strategies for professional development: Transcendental Meditation reduces compassion fatigue and improves resilience for nurses. *Journal for Nurses in Professional Development, 35*(2), 93-97.

Reference 2: Bonamer, J., Kutash, M., Hartranft, S., Aquino-Russell, C., Bugajski, A. & Johnson, A. (2024, in press). Clinical Nurse Well-Being Improved through Transcendental Meditation: A Multi-Method Randomized Controlled Trial. *Journal of Nursing Administration.*

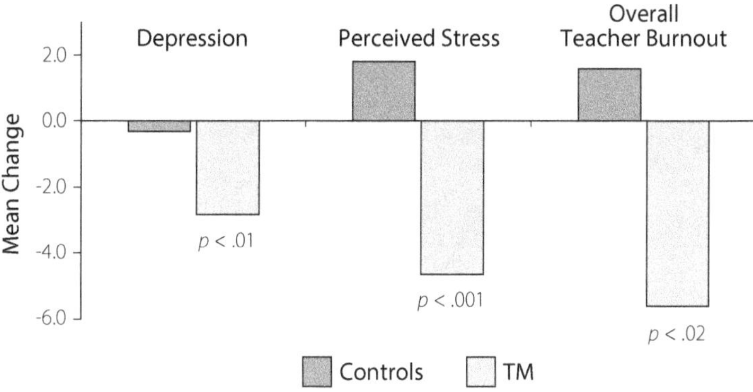

TM decreases depression, stress, and burnout in teachers.

CALM, COLLECTED, EFFECTIVE

"Burnout" is a syndrome of emotional exhaustion, negative attitudes toward others, and dissatisfaction with one's job performance. It is associated with increased absenteeism and job turnover, alcohol and drug abuse, and lower job performance. Workplace stress and burnout are pervasive problems, affecting employee performance and personal health. The issue is thus of importance not only to employers but also to healthcare professionals.

Schoolteachers are among the professionals who may experience a tremendous amount of stress in their work environment. Research indicates that approximately 70% of teachers are under frequent stress, with student discipline problems contributing the most to teacher stress and burnout.

This study of teachers and support staff working in a therapeutic school for students with behavioral problems found that four months of practice of the Transcendental Meditation program significantly reduced depression, how stressed the teachers felt (perceived stress), and overall teacher burnout compared with controls.

The Transcendental Meditation program was effective in reducing psychological distress in teachers. These findings have important implications for employees' job performance as well as their mental and physical health.

Reference: Elder, C., Nidich, S., Moriarty, F., & Nidich, R. (2014). Effect of Transcendental Meditation on employee stress, depression, and burnout: A randomized controlled study. *The Permanente Journal.* 18(1), 19–23.

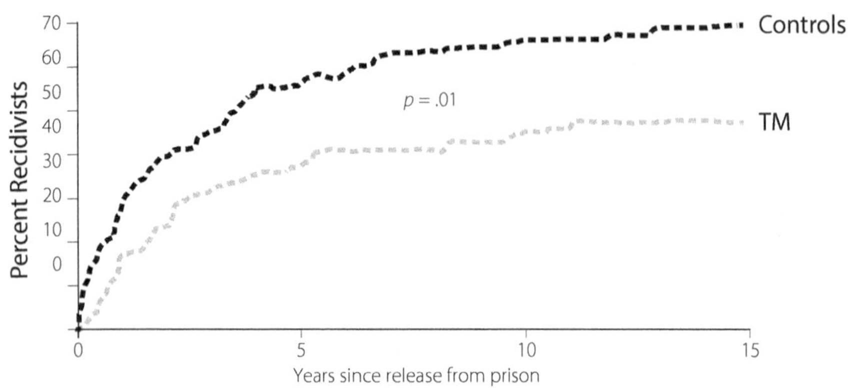

Cumulative proportion over time, of subjects in the TM and Control groups, who were rearrested and reconvicted of felony.

tm-043

LESS RETURN TO PRISON

The chart above shows the results of a followup of prison inmates who had learned the Transcendental Meditation (TM) technique while in prison, for 15 years after they were released. They were parolees, of a maximum security prison in California, who had learned the TM technique while incarcerated. They were compared with controls matched to the TM group on race, offense, prior commitment record, age, and drug use history. Controls had only participated in educational and vocational training or psychotherapy and not in the TM program. The TM group had over 40% fewer re-arrests leading to new felony convictions and new prison terms than controls. (Reference 1)

Similarly, a six-year study compared male felon parolees in three prisons, who learned TM while in prison, with controls matched on parole year, race, institution, and offence, and also compared them with 37,000 statewide parolees. TM parolees had a 46.7% lower reconviction rate than statewide parolees and 30–40% reduced recidivism than controls at five years after release. (Reference 2)

A third study defined recidivism as return to prison for 30 days or more. It was conducted in a maximum security prison in Massachusetts. It found that the TM program reduced recidivism 33% more than four other treatment programs. (Reference 3)

These studies indicate that the TM program is more effective than other programs in reducing recidivism.

Reference 1: Rainforth, M.V., Bleick, C., Alexander, C.N., & Cavanaugh, K.L. (2003). The Transcendental Meditation program and criminal recidivism in Folsom State Prisoners: A 15-year followup study. *Journal of Offender Rehabilitation*, 36, 181–204.

Reference 2: Bleick, C.R., & Abrams, A.I. (1987). The Transcendental Meditation program and criminal recidivism in California. *Journal of Criminal Justice*, 15(3), 211–230.

Reference 3: Alexander, C.N., Rainforth, M.V., Frank, P.R., Grant, J.D., Von Stade, C., & Walton, K.G. (2003). Walpole study of the Transcendental Meditation program in maximum security prisoners III: Reduced recidivism. *Journal of Offender Rehabilitation*, 36(3), 161–180.

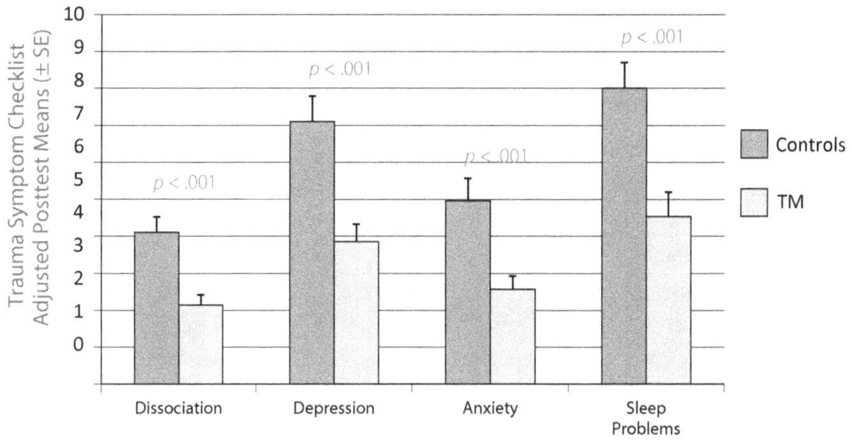

tm-044

DECREASED STRESS & TRAUMA

Prisoners have among the highest rates of lifetime trauma of any segment of society, with recent surveys showing that 85% have been a victim of a crime-related event, such as robbery or home invasion, or physical or sexual abuse. Trauma is associated with higher rates of recidivism (returning to prison) and mental and physical health conditions, including cardiovascular disease.

This study randomly assigned 181 male state correctional inmates to either practice the Transcendental Meditation (TM) program or to be in a control group that only received the prison's usual treatment programs. Compared to controls, the TM group significantly decreased the different dimensions of trauma: anxiety (-48%), depression (-46%), dissociation (-48%), and sleep disturbances (-43%). Reduced dissociation means reduced conflicts between how people feel and think about themselves and their relationships with others. (Reference 1) It indicates that TM increases the integration and wholeness of the personality.

Other controlled studies of prison inmates have found that TM reduces symptoms of schizophrenia and aggression, and unfreezes delayed emotional and personal development. The study found that TM subjects progressed from the "conformist" level where they only thought about themselves in the here and now and were not mindful of the consequences of their behaviors, to the "Self aware" stage where they were more aware of what others think and feel, and thought about the consequences of what they were doing before they acted. In a one-year longitudinal study, inmates who were already practicing TM found that they moved to the "conscientious" stage, corresponding to a more mature and responsible form of cognitive processing, the highest level of personality development typically obtained in adults. (Reference 2)

Reference 1: Nidich, S., O'Connor, T., Rutledge, T., Duncan, J., Compton, B., Seng, A., & Nidich, R. (2016). Reduced trauma symptoms and perceived stress in male prison inmates through the Transcendental Meditation program: A randomized controlled trial. *The Permanente Journal*, 20(4), 16-007.

Reference 2: Alexander, C.N., & Orme-Johnson, D.W. (2003). Walpole study of the TM program in maximum security prisoners II: Longitudinal study of development and psychopathology. *Journal of Offender Rehabilitation*, 36(1–4), 127–160.

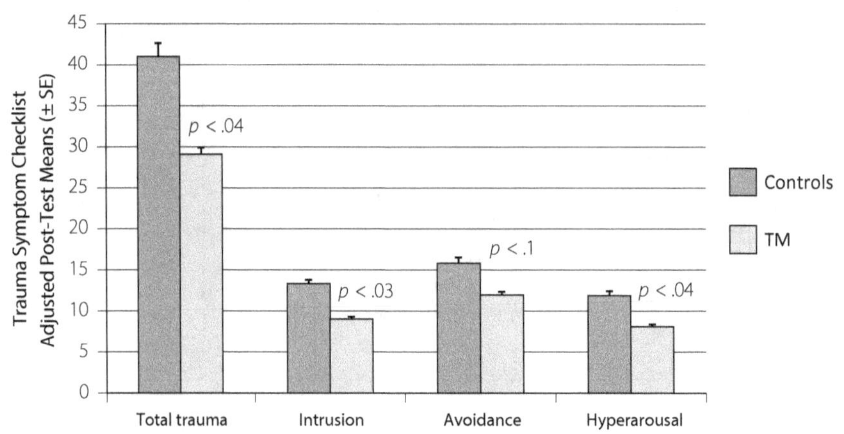

USEFUL THINKING, CALM BEHAVIOR

Past trauma experiences are much higher among incarcerated women compared with the general population.

The objective of this study was to evaluate the effects of the Transcendental Meditation (TM) program on trauma symptoms in female offenders. Inmates at a female correctional facility, with at least 4 months left of incarceration, were enrolled in this randomized controlled study. Subjects were randomly assigned to either the TM group or a wait-list control group.

Subjects were measured at baseline and four-month post-test using the Post-Traumatic Stress Disorder Checklist, which measures intrusive thoughts about the trauma invading the mind, avoidance of things associated with the trauma, and hyperarousal, which means being over-sensitive and jumpy, overreacting to small things.

The study found that compared to controls, the TM group had significant reductions in total trauma, intrusive thoughts, and hyperarousal.

The results of this study indicate the feasibility of the TM program in a female prison population and suggest that TM may be an effective tool for decreasing trauma symptoms.

Reference: Nidich, S., Seng, A., Compton, B., O'Connor, T., Salerno, J.W., & Nidich, R. (2017). Transcendental Meditation and Reduced Trauma Symptoms in Female Inmates: A Randomized Controlled Study. *The Permanente Journal*, 21, 39–43.

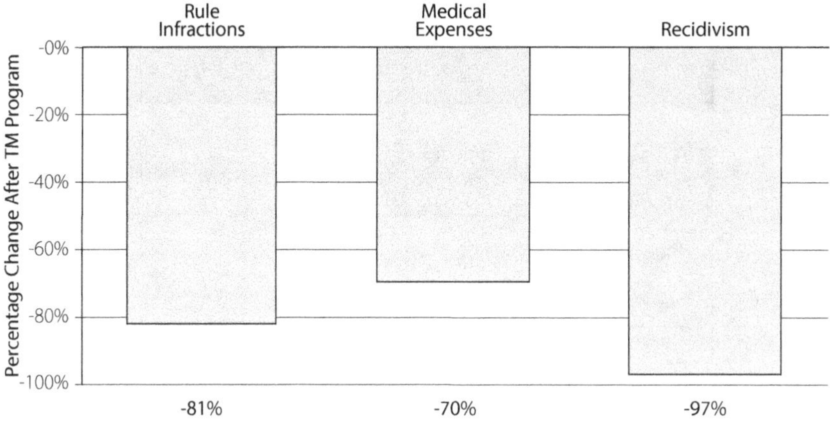

BETTER LIFE INSIDE & OUTSIDE PRISON

Between 1987 and 1989, more than 11,000 inmates and 900 correctional officers and prison administrators in 31 of the 34 prisons in the West African nation of Senegal were instructed in the Transcendental Meditation program. Averaging all 34 prisons (including three where TM was not taught), rule infractions decreased 81% and medical expenses 70%. Among released TM prisoners, recidivism dropped 97%. It is important to note that these results were not the product of a controlled study and, therefore, must be treated with some reserve.

The Senegal project illustrates the significant and positive impact that the use of the Transcendental Meditation program can have on correctional outcomes in prisons in a developing nation. (Reference 1)

Colonel Diop, Director of Penitentiary Administration, made the following comment on the reduction in recidivism in his letter to study organizer and author Mr. Anklesaria: "Considering that there is no structure or scheme for the reintegration of inmates into society, nor is there any provision for work or jobs for those released, it appears that the only possible explanation for this remarkable drop in recidivism in our country is to be found the application of your program." (Anklesaria, January 12, 1989)

Housing fewer people in prison produced a large reduction in the costs of the prison system. Magill's analysis of projected cost savings from TM, working from data on US prison studies, found the overall ratio of program cost to total savings to be at least 1 to 10, with 46% of savings accruing to the correctional system and 54% to the general public. (Reference 2)

Reference 1: Anklesaria, F.K., & King, M.S. (2003). The Transcendental Meditation Program in the Senegalese Penitentiary System. *Journal of Offender Rehabilitation*, 36(1-4), 303-318.

Reference 2: Magill, D.L. (2003). Cost Savings from Teaching the Transcendental Meditation Program in Prisons. *Transcendental Meditation in Criminal Rehabilitation and Crime Prevention*, The Haworth Press, Inc.

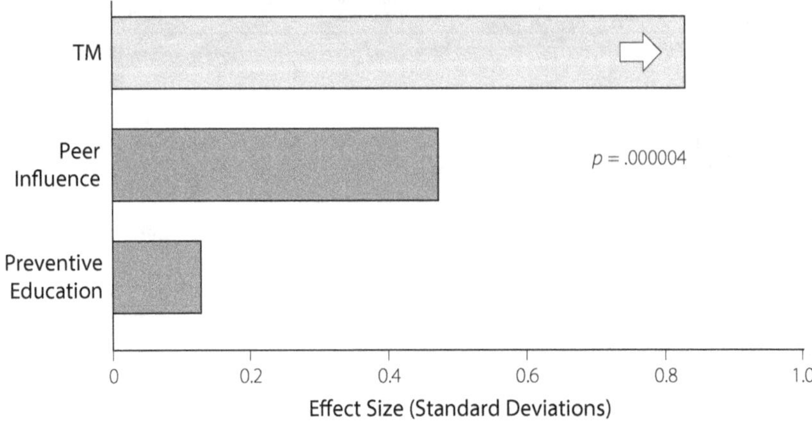

EASIER TO STOP USING DRUGS

People take drugs in an attempt to correct stresses in the body that cause headaches, pain, anxiety, depression, anger, and other symptoms. Research has shown that regular practice of the Transcendental Meditation (TM) technique greatly reduces all these problems and thereby reduces the need for drugs. This is confirmed by this comprehensive meta-analysis, which found that TM was more effective than other treatments available for reducing use of drugs, alcohol, cigarettes, prescribed drugs and non-prescribed illicit drugs.

Typically, for other treatment programs, whether they are for hard drugs, alcohol use, or cigarette consumption, abstinence from use is 100% at the beginning of the program when everyone is inspired for a new start or required to stop using. Sadly, by the end of one year only 10% are still drug-free. For TM, just the opposite is found. Over the course of a year, drug use decreases gradually as regular TM practice normalizes the stresses that provoke this self-medication.

This meta-analysis also found that other relaxation and meditation programs are not as effective as TM.

All meditation practices are not equivalent because other techniques do not provide the uniquely healing state of restful alertness that TM does.

Reference: Alexander, C.N., Robinson, P., & Rainforth, M. (1994). Treating and preventing alcohol, nicotine, and drug abuse through Transcendental Meditation: A review and statistical meta-analysis. *Alcoholism Treatment Quarterly,* 11, 13–88.

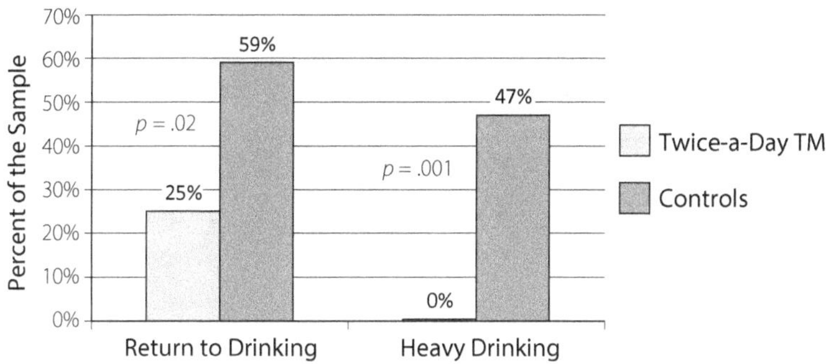

Twice-a-day TM reduces return to drinking after 90 days, and eliminates heavy drinking in patients being treated for alcohol use disorder.

tm-048

REDUCED DRINKING

Adding the Transcendental Meditation (TM) program to other treatments for people undergoing residential rehabilitation for serious Alcohol Use Disorder (AUD) was found to greatly enhance the degree of rehabilitation.

The TM group received Treatment As Usual (TAU), plus TM. The control group received only TAU and included patients doing TM irregularly. The practice of TM twice a day was found to be highly effective for reducing alcohol use. Followup after discharge at 30 days and 90 days found that drinking was markedly reduced in those who usually practiced TM twice a day and that none of the people who practiced TM twice a day returned to heavy drinking.

Maladaptive responses to stress are thought to play a role in addiction and relapse. Relationships between frequency of TM and 3-month outcomes (frequency of alcohol use, heavy drinking, stress, psychological distress, and craving) were examined using Pearson correlations, with confirmation of significant relationships via linear regression, controlling for the baseline value of each outcome.

Integrating TM into inpatient AUD treatment was feasible. Adoption of TM was high (85% doing TM on most of the past 30 days at followup; 61% closely adhering to recommended practice of twice-daily TM). Participants reported high satisfaction with TM.

This study established the feasibility and acceptability of using TM during AUD treatment. Regularly practicing TM (but not just learning it) was consistently associated with better outcomes.

Reference: Gryczynski, J., Schwartz, R.P., Fishman, M.J., Nordeck, C.D., Grant, J., Nidich, S., Rothenberg, S., & E., O.G.K. (2018). Integration of Transcendental Meditation (TM) into alcohol use disorder (AUD) treatment. *Journal of Substance Abuse.*

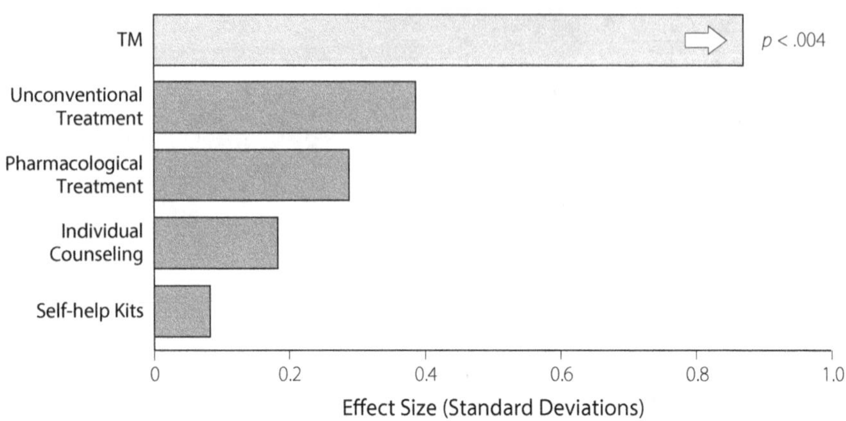

tm-049

EASIER TO KICK THE HABIT

This meta-analysis compared the Transcendental Meditation (TM) technique with published meta-analyses on other standard treatments for smoking cessation.

The primary component of these treatments was one of four intervention types: pharmacological treatment (nicotine replacement therapies, such as nicotine gum); individualized face to face counseling by a physician or counselor; self-help kits consisting of printed material; or unconventional treatments such as acupuncture, relaxation, or hypnosis. The study found that the overall effectiveness of TM on reducing cigarette smoking was 2 to 10 times larger than the other treatment modalities.

The average pre- / post-intervention for TM studies was 12.7 months. Interestingly, the time course of the change due to TM was different from that of standard treatments. For standard treatments, as with other drugs, everyone typically stops smoking at the beginning of the program. But after one year 90% have fallen off and only 10% are not smoking. The TM program does not require a person to stop smoking to learn the technique, but after a year, 90% of the people who have meditated regularly twice a day no longer smoke. This illustrates that the mechanism of TM is gradually normalizing stresses in the physiology that motivate smoking.

As stresses gradually fade away due to self-repair mechanisms of the body normalizing stresses in the unique coherent rest that TM produces, so too does the desire to smoke naturally fade away. This same mechanism has also been found for TM's effects of reducing alcohol and drug usage.

Reference: Alexander, C.N., Robinson, P., & Rainforth, M. (1994). Treating and preventing alcohol, nicotine, and drug abuse through Transcendental Meditation: A review and statistical meta-analysis. *Alcoholism Treatment Quarterly*, 11, 13–88.

Improved Behavior in School

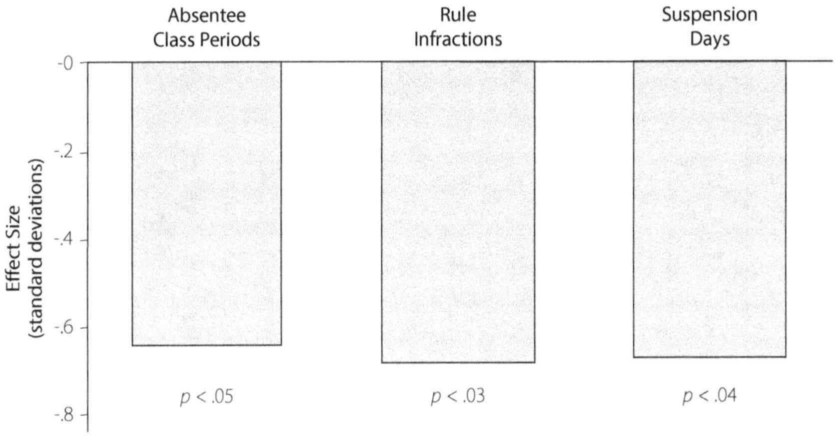

BEHAVE BETTER AT SCHOOL

In this study, inner-city public school adolescent children in the USA were randomly assigned either to learn the Transcendental Meditation (TM) technique or to participate in a health education control group. After four months, the students practicing TM showed decreased absenteeism, fewer school rule infractions, and fewer suspension days. (Reference 1)

In another study conducted in Canada, secondary students who learned TM showed increased tolerance after 14 weeks, in contrast to control students who showed very little improvement. (Reference 2)

Reference 1: Barnes, V.A., Bauza, L.B., & Treiber, F.A. (2003). Impact of stress reduction on negative school behavior in adolescents. *Health Quality Life Outcomes*, 1(1), 10.

Reference 2: Shecter, H.E. (1978). A Psychological Investigation into the Source of the Effect of the TM technique. *Dissertation Abstracts International*, 38(7-B), 3372–3373.

Shecter, H.E. (1977). The Transcendental Meditation Program in the classroom: a psychological evaluation. In Orme-Johnson, D.W. & Farrow, J.T. (Eds.), *Scientific Research on the Transcendental Meditation Program: Collected papers* (Vol. 1). Livingston Manor, New York: Maharishi European University Press (1977).

Decreased Crime in 1% TM Cities in USA

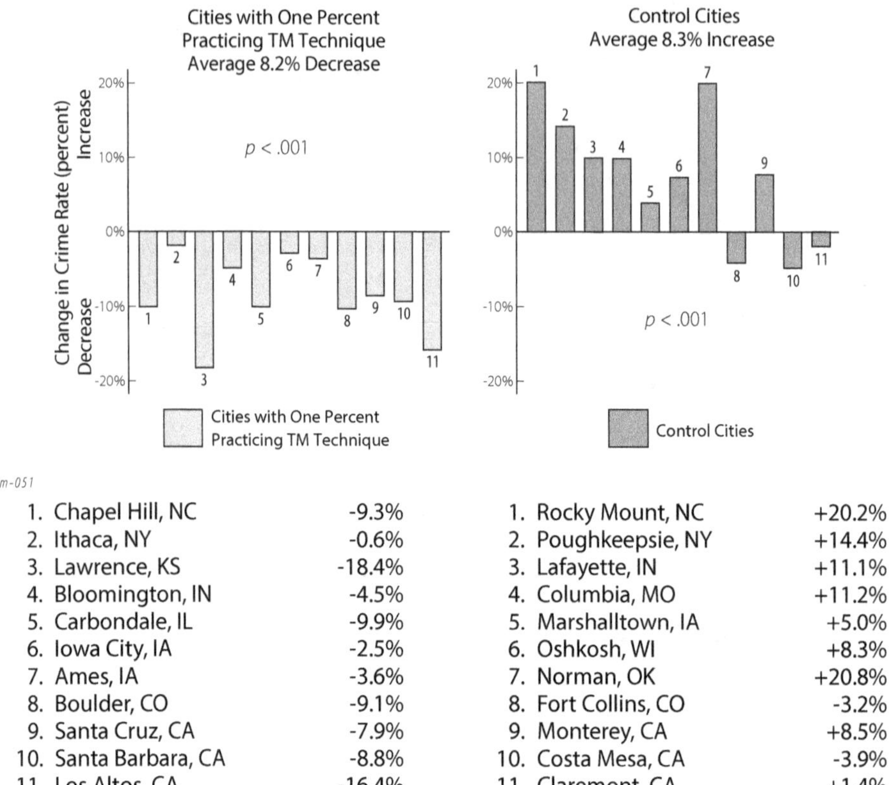

#	Cities with One Percent Practicing TM Technique		#	Control Cities	
1.	Chapel Hill, NC	-9.3%	1.	Rocky Mount, NC	+20.2%
2.	Ithaca, NY	-0.6%	2.	Poughkeepsie, NY	+14.4%
3.	Lawrence, KS	-18.4%	3.	Lafayette, IN	+11.1%
4.	Bloomington, IN	-4.5%	4.	Columbia, MO	+11.2%
5.	Carbondale, IL	-9.9%	5.	Marshalltown, IA	+5.0%
6.	Iowa City, IA	-2.5%	6.	Oshkosh, WI	+8.3%
7.	Ames, IA	-3.6%	7.	Norman, OK	+20.8%
8.	Boulder, CO	-9.1%	8.	Fort Collins, CO	-3.2%
9.	Santa Cruz, CA	-7.9%	9.	Monterey, CA	+8.5%
10.	Santa Barbara, CA	-8.8%	10.	Costa Mesa, CA	-3.9%
11.	Los Altos, CA	-16.4%	11.	Claremont, CA	+1.4%

IMPROVED QUALITY OF CITY LIFE

Decreased Crime in the Environment of Increasing Crime

This study found that in 1975, when 1% or more of a city population learned the Transcendental Meditation (TM) technique, crime rate decreased in those cities. (Reference 1) Moreover, the trend of crime over the following six years decreased in the TM cities compared to matched control cities. (Reference 2)

This was named the Maharishi Effect in honor of Maharishi Mahesh Yogi, who predicted it and provided the technology for its implementation.

Reference 1: Borland, C., & Landrith, G. (1977). Improved quality of Life through the Transcendental Meditation program: Decreased crime rate. In Orme-Johnson, D.W. & Farrow, J.T. (Eds.), *Scientific Research on the Transcendental Meditation Program: Collected papers* (second ed., Vol. 1, pp. 651–658). Maharishi European Research University Press (1977).

Reference 2: Dillbeck, M.C., Landrith III, G., & Orme-Johnson, D.W. (1981). The Transcendental Meditation Program and Crime Rate Changes in a Sample of Forty-Eight Cities. *Journal of Crime and Justice*, 4, 25–45.

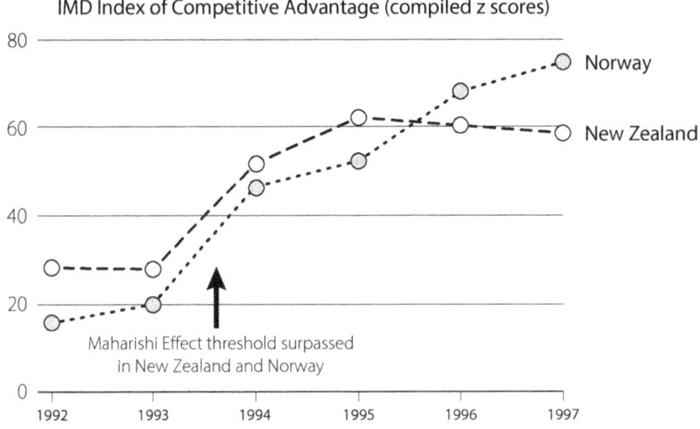

Increased Competitive Advantage in Countries after They Reached 1% of the Population Practicing TM

IMPROVED NATIONAL ECONOMY

Previous research has found that when 1% or more of a city's population begins practicing the Transcendental Meditation (TM) technique, crime in the city decreases and its quality of life improves. (Reference 1) This study extends this finding to the national level of New Zealand and Norway. After reaching the 1% TM threshold, the position of these countries on the Index of National Competitive Advantage increased significantly compared to 44 other developed countries, and continued rising in the following years. Sophisticated mathematical analyses found that the results were not due to statistical artifacts or other factors. The study found that the observed changes were unusually broad-based, sustained, and balanced in nature, with five years of high growth, low unemployment, and low inflation. (Reference 2)

These findings suggest a prescription for balanced and sustained growth, based on a method to enhance quality of life and innovation in the population.

Similar findings have been found in developing nations, including Cambodia and Mozambique. (Reference 3)

Reference 1: Orme-Johnson, D.W., & Fergusson, L. (2018). Global impact of the Maharishi Effect from 1974 to 2017: Theory and Research. *Journal of Maharishi Vedic Research Institute*, 8, 13–76.

Reference 2: Hatchard, G., & Cavanaugh, K.L. (2017). The Effect of Coherent Collective Consciousness on National Quality of Life and Economic Performance Indicators—An Analysis of the IMD Index of National Competitive Advantage. *Journal of Health and Environmental Research*, 3(3-1), 16–31.

Reference 3: Fergusson, L. (2016). The impact of Maharishi Vedic University on Cambodian economic and social indicators from 1980 to 2015. *Journal of Maharishi Vedic Research Institute*, 2, 77–135.

Increased Alpha EEG Coherence During TM
The Basis for Greater Creativity and Learning Ability

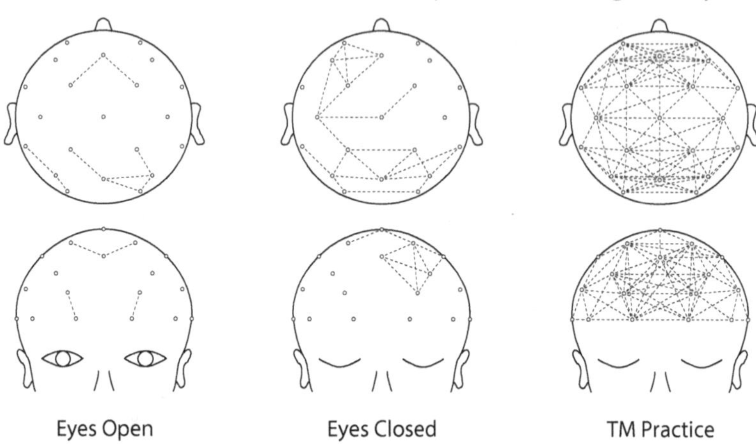

GREATER LEARNING ABILITY & CREATIVITY

During the Transcendental Meditation (TM) technique, the brain works as a unified whole in a state of deep relaxation, as indicated by increased brainwave coherence among all cortical areas, shown in the electroencephalogram (EEG).

The EEG measures electrical activity of the brain ("brainwaves") using electrodes placed on the scalp, as indicated in the illustration above by the dots on the head. Alpha1 EEG seen during TM is a specific frequency of brainwaves (8–10 Hz) which is indicative of restful alertness, when the person is at rest but not drowsy or asleep, and is not engaged in focused activity. Restful alertness is a balanced state of relaxation, yet without focused thinking or problem solving.

During TM, alpha1 EEG increases in power and becomes more coherent, meaning that the brainwaves from different cortical areas begin to function more in phase, as shown by the lines connecting the dots in the illustration. This more harmonious relationship among different parts of the brain that are now working together is called "coherence."

It can be seen in the illustration that although closing the eyes increases coherence (more connecting lines) among just a few areas, TM practice increases coherence much more globally, as indicated by all the dots being connected. (Reference 1)

Higher EEG coherence is associated with decreased anxiety and neuroticism and with increased emotional stability, creativity, intelligence, self-awareness, and moral reasoning. (Reference 2)

Reference 1: *Psychological Bulletin*, 2006, 132(2), 180–211; *Biological Psychology*, 2002, 38(37–51); *Consciousness and Cognition*, 1999, 8(3), 302–318.

Reference 2: *International Journal of Neuroscience*, 1981, 14, 147–151; *International Journal of Neuroscience*, 2006, 116(12), 1519–1538.

Benefits of Coherent Brain Functioning

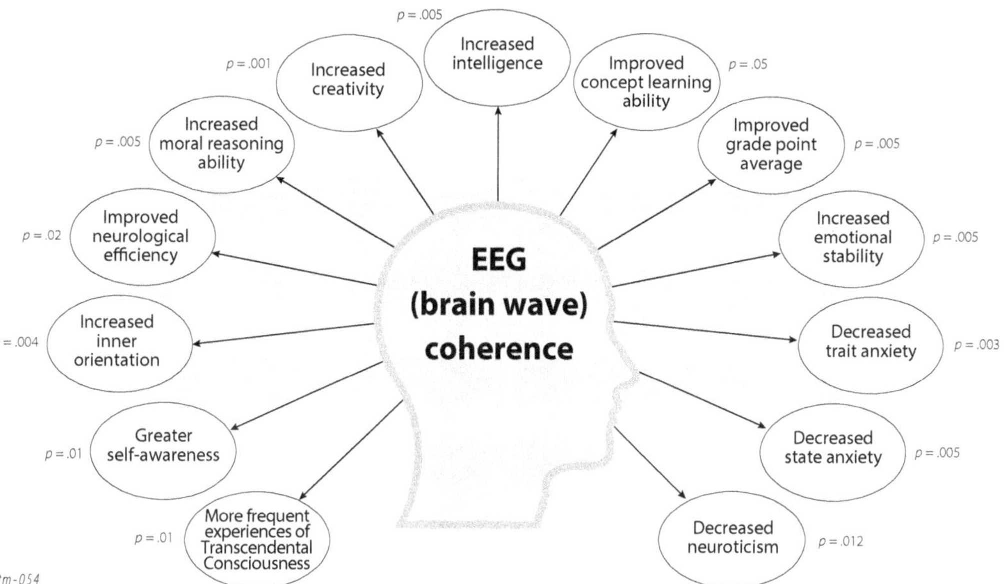

HOLISTIC IMPROVEMENT OF ALL ASPECTS OF LIFE

References:

1. Haynes, C.T., Hebert, R., Reber, W., Orme-Johnson, D.W., The psychophysiology of advanced participants in the Transcendental Meditation program: Correlations of EEG coherence, creativity, H-reflex recovery, and experiences of Transcendental Consciousness. In *Scientific Research on the Transcendental Meditation Program: Collected papers*, Vol. I, edited by Orme-Johnson, D.W., Farrow, J.T., 208–212. Livingston Manor, NY: Maharishi European Research University Press, 1976.

2. Orme-Johnson, D.W., Clements, G., Haynes, C.T., Badawi, K., Higher states of consciousness: EEG coherence, creativity, and experiences of the sidhis. In *Scientific Research on the Transcendental Meditation Program: Collected papers* (Vol. 1), edited by Orme-Johnson, D.W., & Farrow, J. Rheinweiler, Germany: MERU Press, 1977.

3. Travis, F.T., Arenander, A. Cross-sectional and longitudinal study of effects of Transcendental Meditation practice on interhemispheric frontal asymmetry and frontal coherence. *International Journal of Neuroscience* 116, no. 12 (2006): 1519–1538.

4. Orme-Johnson, D.W., Haynes, C.T. EEG phase coherence, pure consciousness, creativity and TM-Sidhi experiences. *International Journal of Neuroscience* 13 (1981): 211–217.

5. Orme-Johnson, D.W., Wallace, R.K., Dillbeck, M.C., et al. Improved functional organization of the brain through the Maharishi Technology of the Unified Field as indicated by changes in EEG coherence and its cognitive correlates. In *Scientific Research on Maharishi's Transcendental Meditation and TM-Sidhi program: Collected papers*, edited by Chalmers, R.A., Clements, G., Schenkluhn, H., Weinless, M., 2245–2266. Vlodrop, The Netherlands: Maharishi Vedic University Press, 1989.

6. Dillbeck, M.C., Orme-Johnson, D.W., Wallace, R.K. Frontal EEG coherence, H-reflex recovery, concept learning, and the TM-Sidhi program. *International Journal of Neuroscience* 15, no. 3 (1981): 151–157.

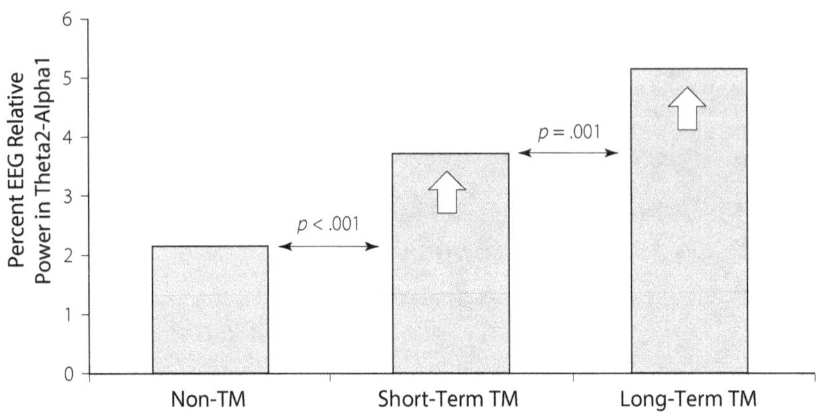

ALL-TIME GOOD MORNING INSIDE

Scientists predicted that if a person were experiencing inner wakefulness during sleep, a sign of Cosmic Consciousness (CC), their EEG would show the EEG of Transcendental Consciousness (TC) simultaneously with the EEG of sleep.

They had previously found that the EEG frequency associated with TC was a frequency band of theta2-alpha1 (6-10 Hz). The EEG signature of deep sleep was well known to be slow waves of 1-4 Hz, called delta.

In contrast to the Short-Term Transcendental Meditation (TM) group or the Non-TM group, during sleep the group reporting signs of Cosmic Consciousness (the Long-Term TM group) had a significantly higher percentage of the theta2-alpha1 EEG of TC, simultaneously with the delta EEG of deep sleep.

The consistent presence of TC during deep sleep would be the conclusive test that Cosmic Consciousness has become fully established in one's physiological functioning.

This experience of the silent inner Self, Transcendental Consciousness or TC, along with sleep or activity is called "witnessing."

This study takes the ancient Vedic knowledge of enlightenment out of the realm of mysticism and into evidence-based modern science, opening the door of enlightenment for everyone.

Reference: Mason, L.I., Alexander, C.N., Travis, F.T., Marsh, G., Orme-Johnson, D.W., Gackenbach, J., et al. Electrophysiological correlates of higher states of consciousness during sleep in long-term practitioners of the Transcendental Meditation program. *Sleep.* 1997 Feb;20(2):102-10.

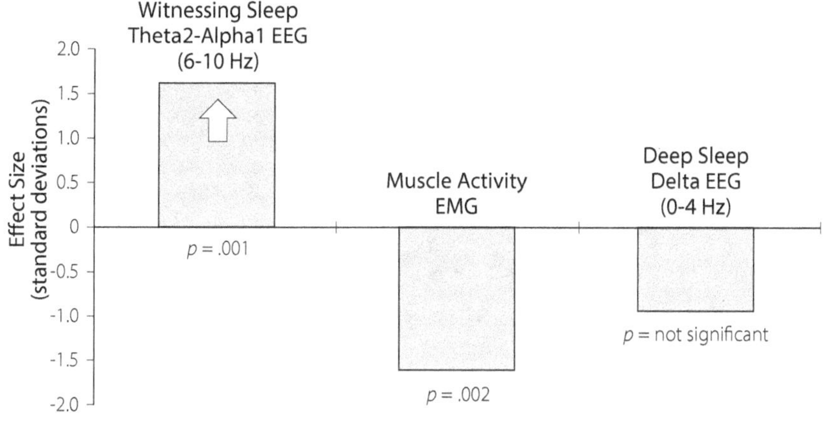

MORE BLISSFUL, RESTFUL SLEEP

One sign of developing Cosmic Consciousness (CC) is the experience of Transcendental Consciousness (TC) during deep sleep—blissful inner awareness, "witnessing." In the chart above, the bars indicate physiological differences between the Long-Term Transcendental Meditation (TM) group, who were witnessing, and the Short-Term TM group, who were not yet experiencing witnessing.

The first bar shows that the Long-Term TM group had more theta2-alpha1 (6-10 Hz), the EEG associated with the experience of Transcendental Consciousness. This indicates that witnessing is based on brain function and is not just subjective.

The second bar shows that during sleep the Long-Term TM group had a greater reduction of electromyography (EMG, muscle activity) during sleep, indicating more relaxed sleep. The third bar shows that the Long-Term TM group had a normal amount of restorative deep "delta" sleep. Their deep sleep was not significantly different from the Short-Term TM group.

This indicates that witnessing sleep is not insomnia, because people with insomnia have fast EEG (associated with thinking), instead of the slower EEGs associated with both normal deep sleep and with Transcendental Consciousness. Insomniacs have restless sleep, not more profound, relaxing sleep.

The unique pattern of brain physiology observed in this experiment corresponds to reports of Cosmic Consciousness in the classical literature on higher states of consciousness throughout the world. It is a developmentally "higher" state of consciousness because research has shown that witnessing is associated with higher levels of moral reasoning, better physical health, and more peak experiences of self-actualization.

Reference: Mason, L.I., Alexander, C.N., Travis, F.T., Marsh, G., Orme-Johnson, D.W., Gackenbach, J., et al. Electrophysiological correlates of higher states of consciousness during sleep in long-term practitioners of the Transcendental Meditation program. *Sleep.* 1997 Feb;20(2):102-10.

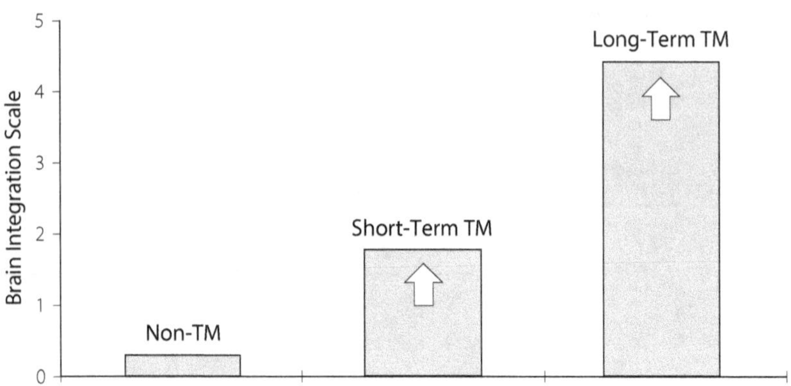

MIND & BODY WORK TOGETHER

This study compared three groups: Long-Term practitioners of the Transcendental Meditation (TM) program who reported witnessing during sleep, a subjective indication of Cosmic Consciousness (CC), and two groups not reporting witnessing at all—Short-Term TMers, and Non-TMers who intended to learn TM.

While awake, during reaction-time tests, Long-Term TMers scored significantly higher on the composite Brain Integration Scale (BIS) than Short-Term TMers and Non-TMers (see chart). They also scored higher on all three BIS factors.

Factor 1: Amplitude of EEG power in the theta2-alpha1 band (6-12 Hz) during activity (the EEG signature of Transcendental Consciousness, present in all areas of the cerebral cortex). The high scores of Long-Term TMers confirm that the subjective experience of witnessing during activity is based on measurable brain function. For the Short-Term TMers and non-TMers, this EEG of witnessing was not found during activity.

Factor 2: Contingent Negative Variation (CNV)—a global cortical brain preparatory response. High scores on this factor indicate that the brain adjusts appropriately to the demands of a situation. When a known specific response is required, the brain mobilizes appropriate perceptual and motor resources to skillfully make that response. If the situation is ambiguous, the high-scoring brain refrains from premature or impulsive action and only moves to respond when it is clear what response is appropriate.

Factor 3: Broadband (6-45 Hz) EEG coherence between the left and right sides of the frontal cortex (the executive brain). High scores indicate focused thinking (beta and gamma, 13-45 Hz) united with Transcendental Consciousness (theta2-alpha1, 6-12 Hz), for increased broad comprehension with the ability to focus sharply. This enables the frontal cortex to express refined emotions, profound reasoning, and an unshakable sense of Self, anchored in pure consciousness.

Reference: Travis, F.T., Tecce, J., Arenander, A., & Wallace, R.K. (2002). Patterns of EEG coherence, power, and contingent negative variation characterize the integration of transcendental and waking states. *Biological Psychology*, 61(293-319).

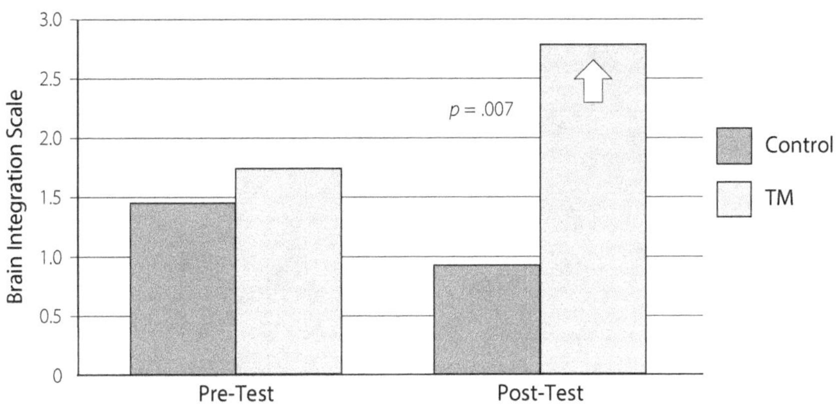

tm-058

INCREASED ORDERLINESS OF BRAIN FUNCTIONING

College student volunteers were randomly assigned to either the Transcendental Meditation (TM) group or a wait-list control group. After testing on both the Brain Integration Scale (BIS) and a stress test, the TM group learned TM and the control group did not. After 10 weeks, both groups were tested again.

The TM group improved 59% on BIS measures of Cosmic Consciousness (CC), whereas the control group decreased by 38% over the same time. This indicates that regular TM increases the development of the orderly style of integrated brain functioning characteristic of Cosmic Consciousness.

The control group probably decreased on the BIS because the post-test was administered during exam week, a very difficult time for most students. This result suggests that stress can *reduce* brain integration as measured by the BIS.

On the stress test, measuring skin conductance responses to loud tones, the control group showed higher levels whereas the TM group stress levels decreased.

The study also found that the TM group decreased in sleepiness, as measured by the Epworth Sleepiness Scale, from pre-test to post-test compared to increased sleepiness among controls.

These results indicate that the progressive integration of Transcendental Consciousness with waking activity through regular TM practice has highly practical benefits for students—increased resistance to stress, more wakefulness, and increased brain integration with its benefits of faster and more accurate decisions, more frequent experiences of self-actualization, and higher levels of moral reasoning.

Reference: Travis, F.T., Haaga, D., Hagelin, J.S., Tanner, M., Nidich, S.I., King, C.G., et al. Effects of Transcendental Meditation practice on brain functioning and stress reactivity in college students. *International Journal of Psychophysiology.* 2009;71(2):170-6.

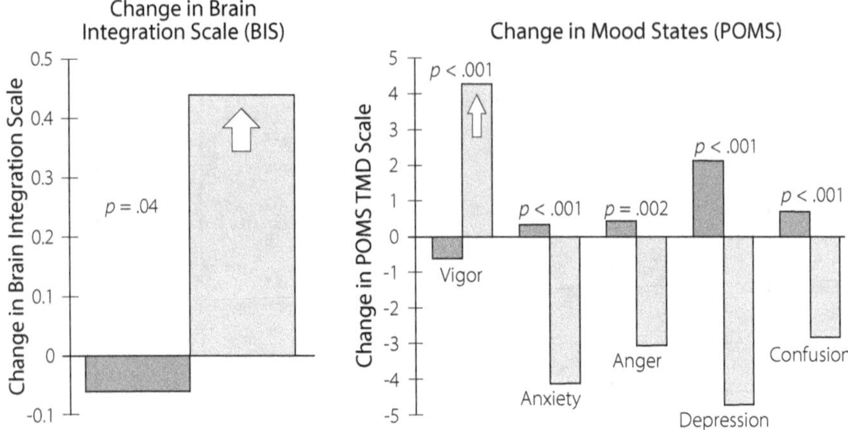

INTEGRATED BRAINS ACCOMPLISH MORE

Ninety-six central office administrators and staff (mean age 46) in a major urban school district were randomly assigned to either start the Transcendental Meditation (TM) program immediately or be in a wait-list control group. At "baseline" (before learning TM), participants completed an online Profile of Mood States questionnaire (POMS). A subset (N=79) also had their EEG recorded to calculate Brain Integration Scale (BIS) scores, which measure progress toward Cosmic Consciousness (Transcendental Consciousness along with activity). The POMS and EEG/BIS recordings were repeated after four months ("post-test").

The left-hand chart shows a significant increase in BIS scores in the EEG of TM participants, indicating growth in the brain physiology of Cosmic Consciousness (CC), which is also found in the brain physiology of the most successful members of society.

The right-hand bar chart shows a significant decrease on the POMS Total Mood Disturbance scale, and on the anxiety, anger, depression, fatigue, and confusion subscales, along with a significant increase on the POMS vigor subscale.

Rising scores in the BIS, with greater vigor and decreased anxiety, anger, depression, and confusion, confirm that these changes in how the brain is working underlie the greater energy and effectiveness in life experienced with growth of CC.

The practical value of growth toward CC is that action no longer arises from narrow self-interest, fears, and pre-judgments (prejudices). In CC, action arises from a more holistic appreciation of the situation, because Transcendental Consciousness is the home of all the laws of nature. Action is more vigorous and productive because inner resistance and confusion no longer interfere with decision-making and action. The brain waits for all relevant information before it acts, and then coordinates more skills and capabilities to accomplish any particular task.

Compliance with TM practice was high (93%), indicating that the administrators and staff enjoyed their TM program.

Reference: Travis, F., Valosek, L., Konrad, A., Link, J., Salerno, J., Scheller, R., & Nidich, S. (2018). Effect of meditation on psychological distress and brain functioning: A randomized controlled study. *Brain and Cognition*, 125, 100-105.

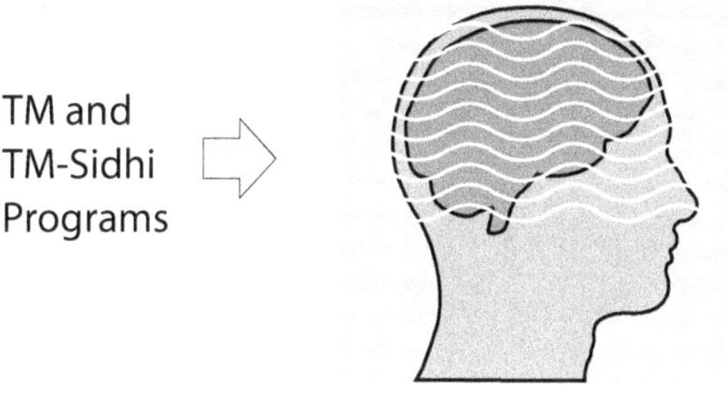

Increased Brain Integration

The TM and TM-Sidhi programs increase brain integration, which is the hallmark of creativity and success in many professions.

tm-060

ACCOMPLISHMENT & SUCCESS

Growth toward Cosmic Consciousness, the first stable state of enlightenment, has been found to be associated with a high level of brain integration. Randomized controlled trials, the most rigorous type of research, found that regular practice of the Transcendental Meditation (TM) technique increases brain integration.

In this study of people *not* practicing TM, top-level managers and world-class athletes scored higher on the Brain Integration Scale (BIS) than less successful peers. The BIS measures coherent functioning in the frontal executive areas of the brain, which coordinate holistic thought and behavior that will be successful in any situation. High BIS scores also indicate restfully alert and efficient brain function. Subjects also scored higher on moral reasoning and self-development, and recovered faster from stress. Even though they had not learned TM, they had more frequent experiences associated with Transcendental Consciousness during waking activity, resting, and sleep; these experiences are classical subjective indicators of Cosmic Consciousness.

Other research showed that police with higher brain integration were more spiritual and were better than other police in throwing off the stress of police work before entering back into their family life. World class musicians, compared to less-skilled musicians, had greater cognitive flexibility, faster brain processing, higher levels of moral reasoning, and more frequent transcendental experiences. However, both levels of musicians had high measures of brain integration, supporting other research which showed that learning to play a musical instrument is good for your brain.

Research has also found that higher BIS scores are correlated with standard measures of originality, flexibility, and fluency of creative thought. TM practice increases this coherence and research confirms that this coherence is found in more successful people. This helps explain why TM leads to more success in life.

References: Harung, H., & Travis, F. (2011). Higher mind-brain development in successful leaders: testing a unified theory of performance. *Cognitive Processing*, 13(2), 171-181.

Harung, H., & Travis, F. (2019). *World-Class Brain: The edge that helps peak performers succeed and how you can develop it*. Harvest AS.

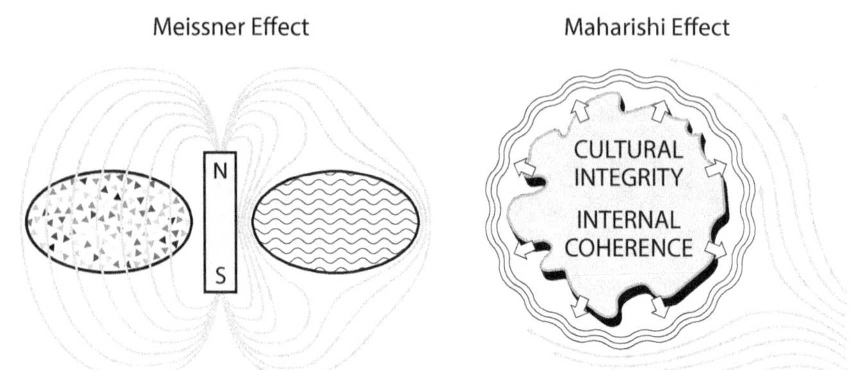

tm-061

INNER & OUTER INVINCIBILITY

The Meissner Effect documents an example from nature of how invincibility can work in physical systems.

These classic experiments are illustrated in the left portion of the chart above. A magnet in the center creates a field of magnetic waves that typically would penetrate all the objects around it.

The diagram shows an ordinary conductor (left of the magnet), whose incoherence or disordered electrons are easily penetrated by the magnetic field, shown by the magnetic field lines crossing over (and disrupting) the area of disorganized dots. On the right of the magnet, we see a coherent collective state of high-order electron flow, which rejects external magnetic influence and thus makes the conductor impenetrable, shown by the magnetic field lines bending around the area of coherence.

The right portion of the chart illustrates a nation with sufficient people coherent enough to create a national field of coherence strong enough to repel disorderly influences and maintain cultural integrity and invincibility.

Individual Invincibility. As individuals heal their stress and fatigue, and grow in the direction of enlightenment through regular practice of the Transcendental Meditation (TM) technique, they become established in Transcendental Consciousness (TC), the unshakable experience of bliss and inner light at the foundation of the mind. On the basis of this inner stability and clarity of mind, they become masters of their fate, no longer at the mercy of situations and circumstances. They are "freed from duality, ever firm in purity, independent of possessions, possessed of the Self" (*Bhagavad-Gita*, 2.45); in a word, invincible.

National Invincibility. As the people in a nation rise to enlightenment, the influence of coherence they generate in collective consciousness helps society to maintain internal harmony and integrity. It provides a national armor, an invisible border which makes the nation impenetrable to harmful influences from outside, promoting cultural integrity and progress. This is called the "Maharishi Effect."

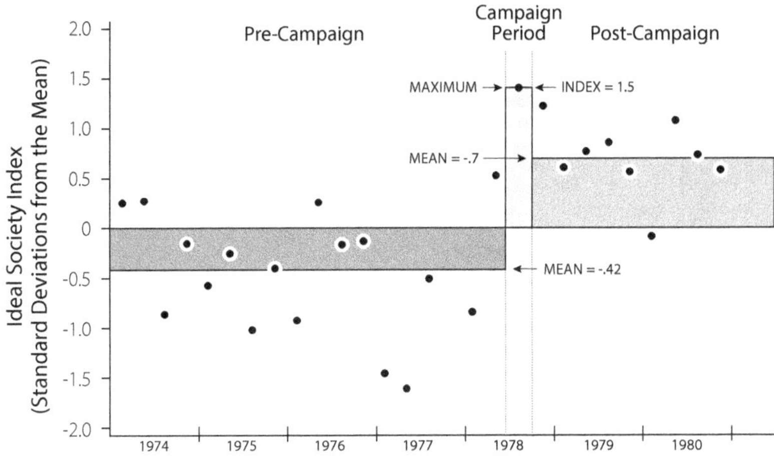

DISCOVERY OF THE √1% EFFECT

When the Transcendental Meditation (TM) teachers meditated together in groups in Rhode Island in 1978 during the Ideal Society Campaign, the Ideal Society Index rose to a maximum of 1.5 (see Campaign Period in the chart above). This was significantly higher than the mean of –.42 for the five year Pre-Campaign. (See Pre-Campaign period in chart. Dots show data points and gray area indicates the mean.) The rise in the Ideal Society Index during the campaign indicates large, highly significant decreases in the composite index of crimes, deaths, motor accidents and fatalities, unemployment, pollution, and consumption of alcohol ($p < .0005$).

Moreover, after the TM teachers left the state, during the three-year Post-Campaign period the mean of the Ideal Society Index settled to .7, which is still significantly higher than during the Pre-Campaign period ($p < .0005$). This reflects that the TM teachers were successful in teaching enough people the TM technique to have a lasting effect on maintaining a higher quality of life in the state.

This discovery led to the √1% formula—√1% of a population practicing the TM-Sidhi program together is sufficient to produce the Maharishi Effect.

This reduced requirement opened the possibility of creating relatively small groups of TM-Sidhi participants to have a predicted positive effect on the trends of time in populations of any size—city, state, national, or world. Subsequent research has confirmed this prediction on all these levels.

References: Dillbeck, M.C., Cavanaugh, K.L., Glenn, T., Orme-Johnson, D.W., & Mittlefehldt, V. (1987). Consciousness as a Field: The Transcendental Meditation and TM-Sidhi Program and Changes in Social Indicators. *The Journal of Mind and Behavior*, 8(1), 67–104.

Dillbeck, M.C., Foss, A., & Zimmermann, W. (1989). Maharishi's Global Ideal Society Campaign: Improved quality of life in Rhode Island through the Transcendental Meditation and TM-Sidhi program. In R. Chalmers, G. Clements, H. Schenkluhn, & M. Weinless (Eds.), *Scientific research on Maharishi's Transcendental Meditation and TM-Sidhi program: Collected papers*, Vol. 4. Maharishi Vedic University Press.

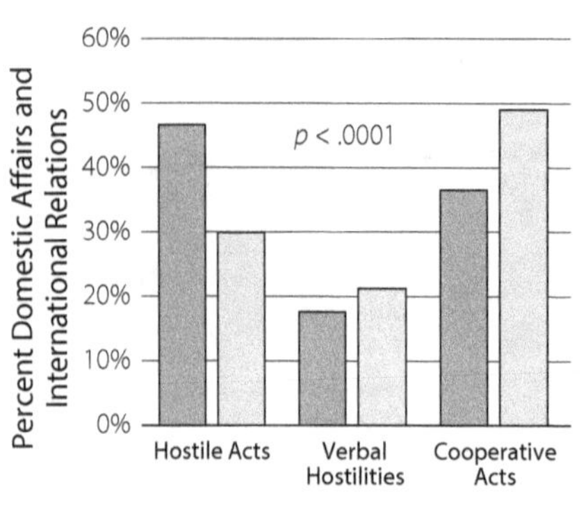

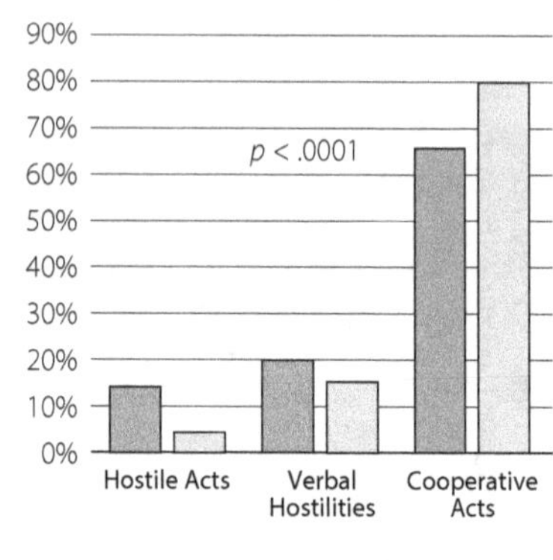

tm-063

LESS WAR, MORE PEACE

During the World Peace Project, news reports from the trouble-spot countries, as well as from the USA, Russia, and other major nations, reported an unexpected wave of restored balance to the socio-political systems in those areas and in the world. (Reference 1)

The World Peace Project, bringing groups doing the Transcendental Meditation (TM) and TM-Sidhi program to trouble-spots in the world, was formally evaluated using data on international and domestic conflicts recorded in the Conflict and Peace Data Bank (COPDAB) file, which contains 14,567 events for 1978.

Within the trouble-spot countries, during the 10-week period of the project (October 8 – December 23, 1978), compared to the 10-week baseline period before the project, there were significant decreases in hostile acts of war and increases in cooperative activities, such as economic, technological, and cultural exchanges.

Worldwide, the level of hostilities was much lower and cooperation higher than in the trouble spots. And during the World Peace Project, hostilities decreased further and cooperation increased. It is interesting to note that during the World Peace Project there was an increase in verbal hostility, suggesting that some of the physical violence downgraded into verbal abuse. Worldwide, verbal hostilities also decreased.

Comparing what happened in 1978 with the prior 10-year period showed that violence did not decrease at that time of year in previous years, controlling for year-end effects and holidays. (Reference 2)

Reference 1: Maharishi Mahesh Yogi. (1979). The Dawn of World Peace: The Responsibility of All Peoples and Governments. *World Government of the Age of Enlightenment*, Issue 11.

Reference 2: Orme-Johnson, D.W., Dillbeck, M.C., Bousquet, J.G., & Alexander, C.N. (1979). The World Peace Project of 1978: An experimental analysis of the application of the Maharishi Technology of the Unified Field in major world trouble spots: Increased harmony in international affairs. In Chalmers, R.A., Clements, G., Schenkluhn, H., & Weinless, M. (Eds.), *Scientific Research on Maharishi's Transcendental Meditation and TM-Sidhi program: Collected papers*, Vol. 4 Vlodrop (pp. 2532–2548). Maharishi Vedic University Press.

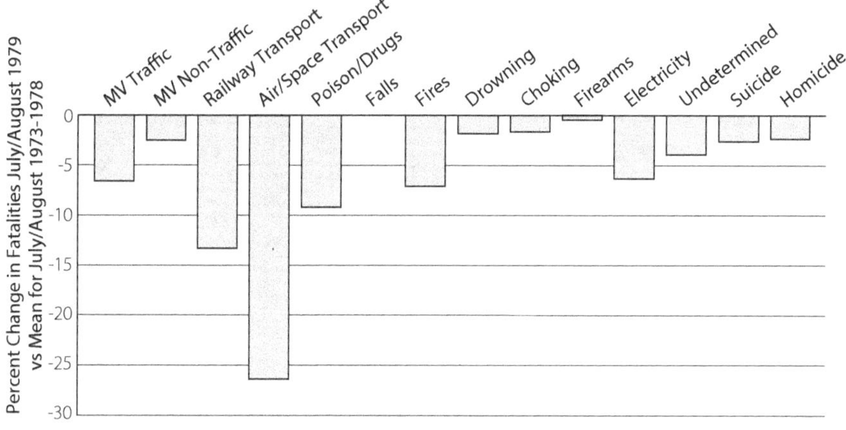

THE FIRST WORLD PEACE ASSEMBLY

Based on prior research and theory, this study tested two predictions: 1) that the group of 2500 Transcendental Meditation (TM) and TM-Sidhi program participants assembled in Amherst MA in the summer of 1979 would improve the quality of life in the United States, and 2) that the effects would be even greater in the state of Massachusetts where the group was located.

As predicted, compared with levels expected for the same period over the years 1973–1978, there were significant reductions for the USA, during the six-week experimental period, in motor vehicle (MV) fatalities, violent crimes, air transport fatal accidents, and consistently across the 14 major independent categories of fatal accidents shown above. At the same time, the Standard and Poor's and the Dow Jones stock indices increased significantly compared to prior trends.

Also, as predicted, improvements in and near the state of Massachusetts were significantly greater than those for the rest of the USA. For example, for the New England region, motor vehicle fatalities were down by 18.9%, violent crimes by 10.1%, and air transport fatal accidents by 83.3%, compared to lesser changes in the USA as a whole.

The consistent improvements across a broad range of independent indices of social order, and across geographical areas, during the experimental period, are most simply explained in terms of enhanced coherence in an underlying field of collective consciousness both in the USA as a whole, and within Massachusetts, through the collective practice of the Maharishi Technology of the Unified Field.

Reference. Davies, J.L., & Alexander, C.N. (1983/1989). The Maharishi Technology of the Unified Field and improved quality of life in the United States: A study of the First World Peace Assembly, Amherst, Massachusetts, 1979. In Chalmers, R.A., Clements, G., Schenkluhn, G., & Weinless, M. (Eds.), *Scientific Research on Maharishi's Transcendental Meditation and TM-Sidhi program: Collected papers* (Vol. 4). Maharishi Vedic University Press.

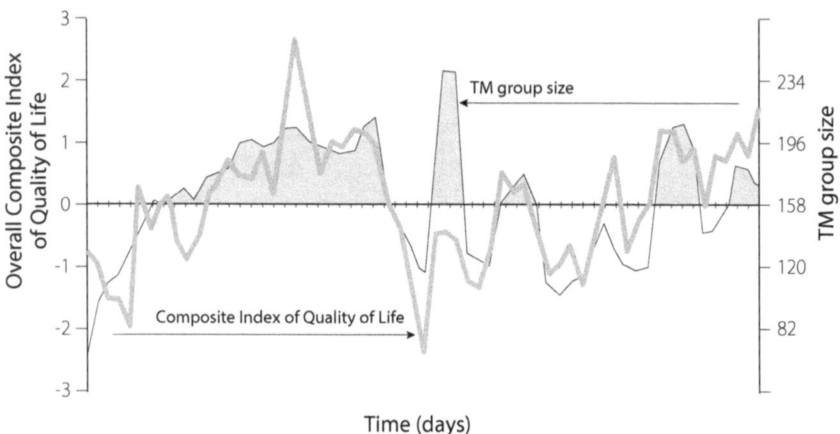

COHERENCE GROUP IN JERUSALEM
HELPS ISRAEL & LEBANON

Increasing numbers of participants in Maharishi's Transcendental Meditation (TM) and TM-Sidhi program in a group located in Jerusalem led to improved quality of life in Israel and Lebanon. The chart shows a strong correspondence between the number of TM-Sidhi participants and a composite index of quality of life comprising many variables, including war intensity and war deaths in Lebanon, Israeli national stock market prices and national mood, and auto accident rates, number of fires, and crime rates in Jerusalem and Israel.

Reference: Orme-Johnson, D.W., Alexander, C.N., Davies, J.L., Chandler, H.M., & Larimore, W.E. (1988). International Peace Project: The Effects of the Maharishi Technology of the Unified Field. *Journal of Conflict Resolution*, 32(4), 776–812.

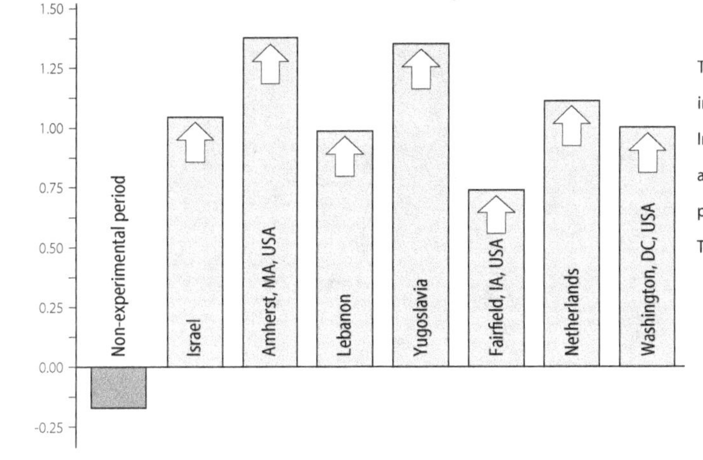

GROUPS AT A DISTANCE
CREATE PEACE IN LEBANON

The results of reduced war in Lebanon during the International Peace Project, which brought groups practicing the Transcendental Meditation (TM) and TM-Sidhi program to the Middle East, were subsequently replicated in seven consecutive experiments over a two-year period during the peak of the Lebanon war. The results of these interventions included:

- War-related fatalities decreased by 71% ($p < 10^{-10}$) (less than 1 in one billion).

- War-related injuries fell by 68% ($p < 10^{-6}$) (less than 1 in one million).

- The level of conflict dropped by 48% ($p < 10^{-8}$) (less than 1 in one hundred million).

- Cooperation among antagonists increased by 66% ($p < 10^{-6}$) (less than 1 in one million).

The likelihood that these combined results were due to chance or other factors is less than one in 10^{-19} (1 in 1,000,000,000,000,000,000, or 1 in one quadrillion). This level of statistical significance establishes that the Maharishi Effect—of reducing societal stress and violence by the establishment of a coherence-creating group practicing the TM and TM-Sidhi program—is one of the most rigorously established phenomena in the history of the social sciences.

Reference: Davies, J.L., & Alexander, C.N. (2005). Alleviating political violence through reducing collective tension: Impact assessment analysis of the Lebanon war. *Journal of Social Behavior and Personality*, 17(1), 285–338.

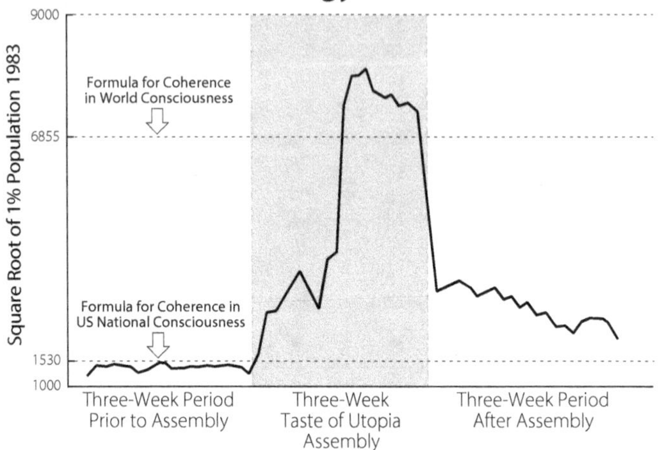

THE MAHARISHI EFFECT IN NATIONAL
& WORLD CONSCIOUSNESS

When the Taste of Utopia Assembly began on December 17, 1983, the size of the existing coherence-creating group at MIU increased to more than 6,855, the square root of one percent of the world's population in 1983. The threshold for affecting national and world consciousness was reached, as can be seen in the graph above.

On January 6, 1984 the Taste of Utopia Assembly ended and the number of people practicing the Transcendental Meditation (TM) and TM-Sidhi program together fell far below the Maharishi Effect threshold, the number needed to maintain coherence and positivity in world consciousness. This change marked the end of the Assembly time period.

During this Utopia Assembly Period, the world experienced healthier world economy, more prosperity world-wide, reduced crime, reduced traffic and air-traffic fatalities, increased national creativity, more effective heads of state, and less international conflict.

Reference: Orme-Johnson, D.W., Cavanaugh, K.L., Alexander, C.N., Gelderloos, P., Dillbeck, M.C., Lanford, A., & Abou Nader, T.M. (1984). The influence of the Maharishi Technology of the Unified Field on world events and global social indicators: The effects of the Taste of Utopia assembly. In Chalmers, R., Clements, G., Schenkluhn, H., & Weinless, M. (Eds.), *Scientific Research on Maharishi's Transcendental Meditation and TM-Sidhi Program: Collected papers (Vol. 4)*. Maharishi Vedic University Press.

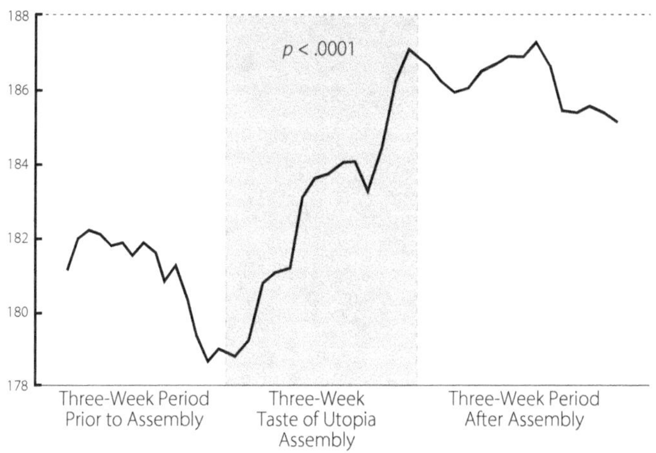

HEALTHIER WORLD ECONOMY

In the three weeks prior to the Taste of Utopia Assembly, the World Index of stock prices was declining. However, this declining trend was reversed as soon as the size of the Assembly began to increase, and the stock markets increased proportionately. This indicates that the Utopia Assembly created a global wave of confidence and optimism in the economic health of the financial markets. After the Utopia Assembly ended, abruptly decreasing the size of the coherence-creating group, the world stock markets began to waver and then began a declining trend similar to the trend prior to the Utopia Assembly.

Careful analysis of market dynamics in previous years showed that they do not typically increase at this time of year, nor could the increase in the world stock markets be attributed to anything else that might be happening at that time.

Reference: *Scientific Research on Maharishi's Transcendental Meditation and TM-Sidhi Program: Collected papers, (Vol. 4).* 1984: 2730-2762.

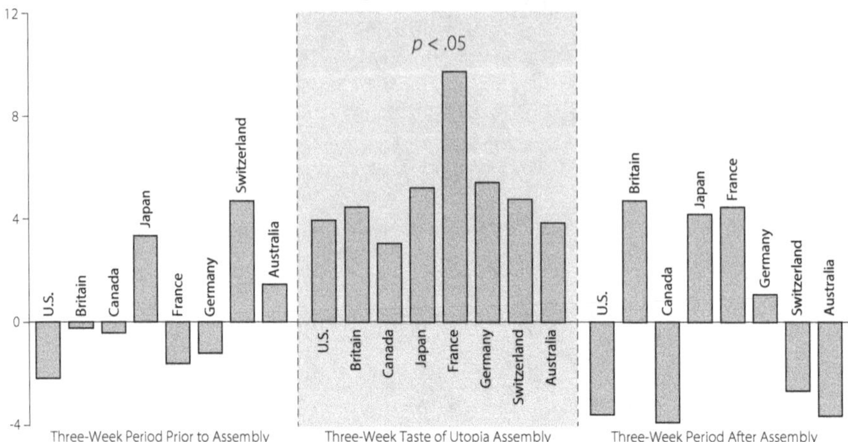

MORE PROSPERITY WORLDWIDE

During the Taste of Utopia Assembly, the major stock markets of the world increased simultaneously, indicating balanced economic growth worldwide.

After the Assembly, the same major stock markets reverted to a pattern similar to that seen prior to the Assembly, with some increasing and some decreasing.

Reference: *Scientific Research on Maharishi's Transcendental Meditation and TM-Sidhi Program: Collected papers, (Vol. 4).* 1984: 2730-2762.
Data source: Capital International SA, Geneva (*Wall Street Journal*)

Percent Change in Daily or Weekly Crime Totals

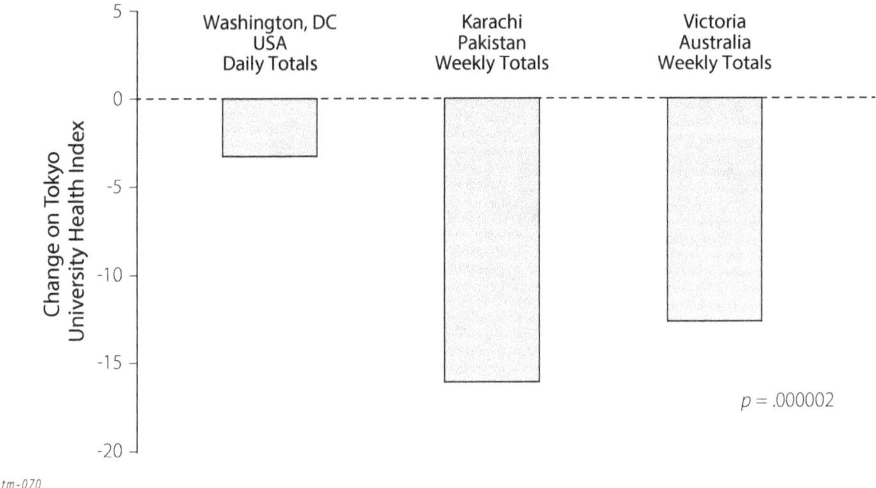

REDUCED CRIME

Using time series analysis it was found that during the Taste of Utopia Assembly, significant decreases occurred in daily or weekly crime totals, in locations on three continents, in comparison with the average daily or weekly totals for the 24 weeks prior to, and 3 weeks after, the Assembly.

Reference: *Scientific Research on Maharishi's Transcendental Meditation and TM-Sidhi Program: Collected papers, (Vol. 4).* 1984: 2730-2762.

Data sources: City Police Department, Washington, DC; Inspector-General of Police, Government of Sind, Karachi, Islamic Republic of Pakistan; Research and Development Department, Victoria Police, Melbourne, Australia.

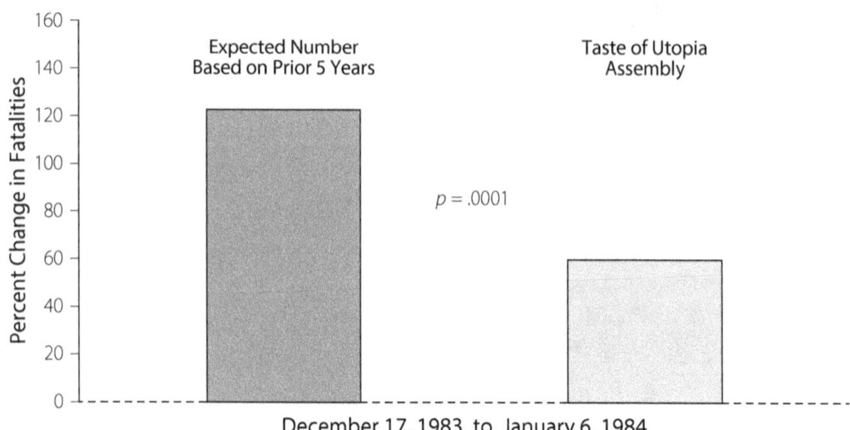

WORLDWIDE DECREASE
IN AIR TRAFFIC FATALITIES

During the Taste of Utopia Assembly the number of air traffic fatalities in the world was 49% lower than the expected number, based on the prior five years for the same time of year. It was also 29% lower than the lowest number during the equivalent three-week period in the prior five years.

Reference: *Scientific Research on Maharishi's Transcendental Meditation and TM-Sidhi Program: Collected papers, (Vol. 4). 1984: 2730-2762.*
Data sources: International Civil Aviation Organization; National Transportation Safety Board, USA.

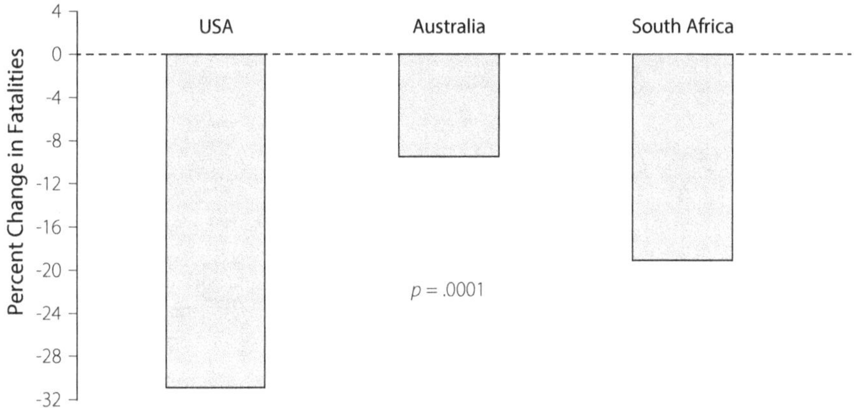

DECREASED TRAFFIC FATALITIES

Traffic fatalities decreased significantly during the Taste of Utopia Assembly. In the USA, traffic fatalities per day over the Christmas and New Year's weekends were at an all-time low, even though, despite the cold weather, miles driven per day were at an all-time high.

Reference: *Scientific Research on Maharishi's Transcendental Meditation and TM-Sidhi Program: Collected papers, (Vol. 4).* 1984: 2730-2762.
Data sources: National Safety Council, USA; National Road Safety Council, South Africa; and in Australia, State Police Dept., Sydney; Police Dept., Perth; and Road Traffic Authority, Hawthorn. [Note: Traffic fatalities for Australia are for Western Australia, New South Wales, and Victoria.]

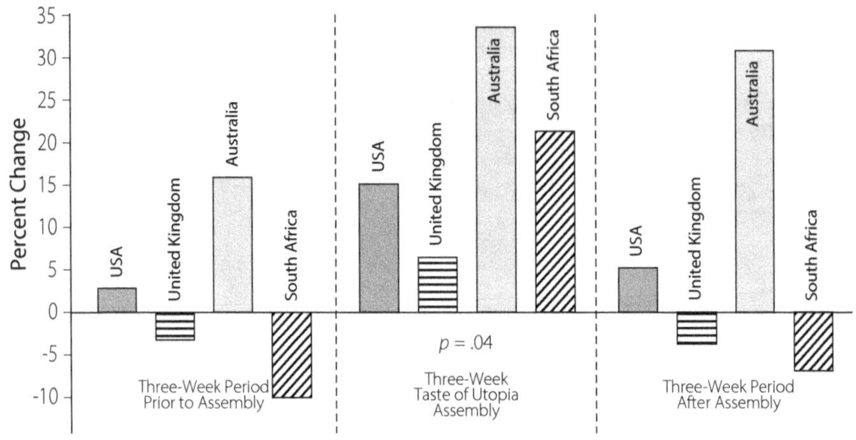

INCREASED NATIONAL CREATIVITY

During the Taste of Utopia Assembly the number of patents filed, an important measure of national creativity, increased significantly in countries on four continents. After the Assembly, the number of applications tended to revert to a pattern similar to that seen prior to the Assembly.

Reference: *Scientific Research on Maharishi's Transcendental Meditation and TM-Sidhi Program: Collected papers, (Vol. 4).* 1984: 2730-2762.
Data sources: US Patent Office; UK Patent Office; Australia Patent, Trade Marks, and Design Office; Government Patent Office, South Africa.

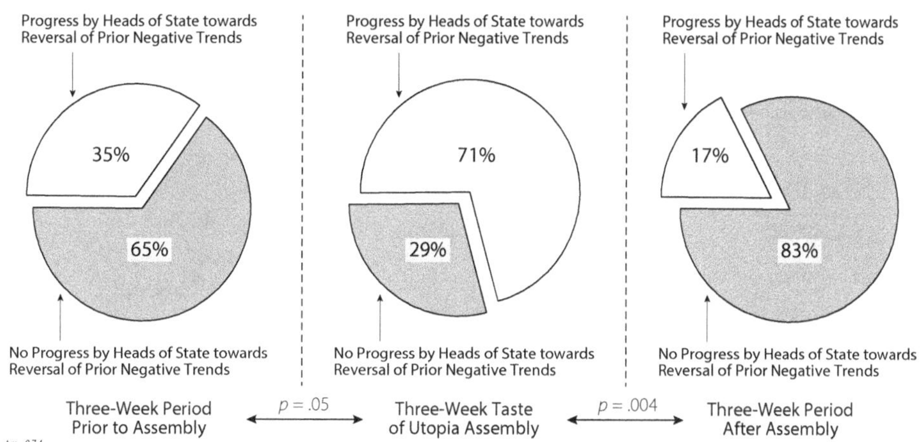

MORE EFFECTIVE HEADS OF STATE

According to Maharishi's Absolute Theory of Government, government is the innocent mirror of the nation, and the head of state reflects by their speech and actions the quality of national consciousness. During the Taste of Utopia Assembly, coherence increased in world consciousness as exhibited by more positive, evolutionary statements and actions of heads of state of nations throughout the world, and by more national and international support for their policies and leadership.

After the Assembly the quality of the statements and actions of heads of state, and the support they received, reverted toward less positivity.

Reference: *Scientific Research on Maharishi's Transcendental Meditation and TM-Sidhi Program: Collected papers, (Vol. 4).* 1984: 2730-2762.
Data source: Content analysis from *The New York Times.*

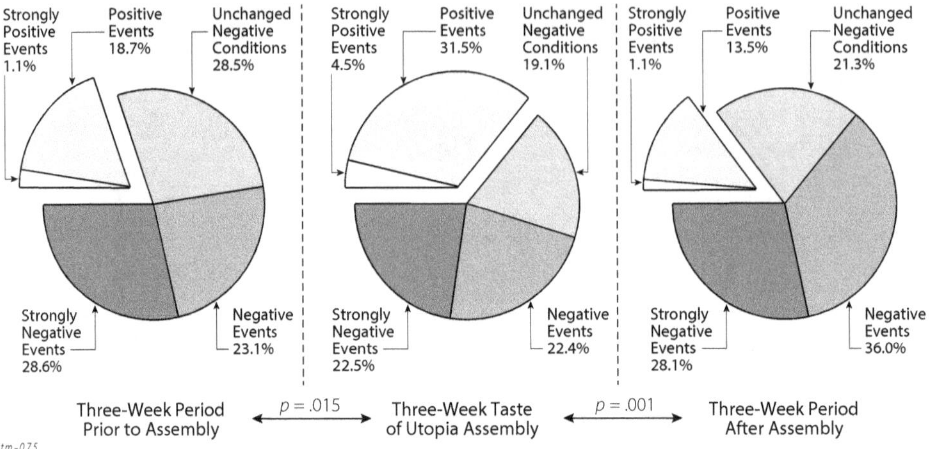

LESS INTERNATIONAL CONFLICT

During the three-week period of the Taste of Utopia Assembly, the balance of negativity to positivity in events pertaining to international conflicts in the trouble-spot areas of the world shifted significantly toward increased positivity.

After the Assembly the balance of events reverted toward increased negativity.

Based on theory and previous research, the hypothesis was publicly announced in advance that single large groups of Transcendental Meditation and TM-Sidhi program participants exceeding the predicted threshold of $\sqrt{1\%}$ of the world population (about 7,000 people at the time) would reduce international conflicts.

On the three occasions when such assemblies were held, international conflicts decreased by about 30% and global terrorism decreased by 72%. The three assemblies were the Taste of Utopia Assembly in Fairfield Iowa, USA, December 1983 to January 1984; Vedic Science Conference, The Hague, The Netherlands, December 1984 to January 1985; and the World Assembly on Vedic Science, Washington, DC, USA, July 1985.

Reference: *Scientific Research on Maharishi's Transcendental Meditation and TM-Sidhi Program: Collected papers, (Vol. 4). 1984: 2730-2762.*
Data source: Content analysis from *The New York Times.*

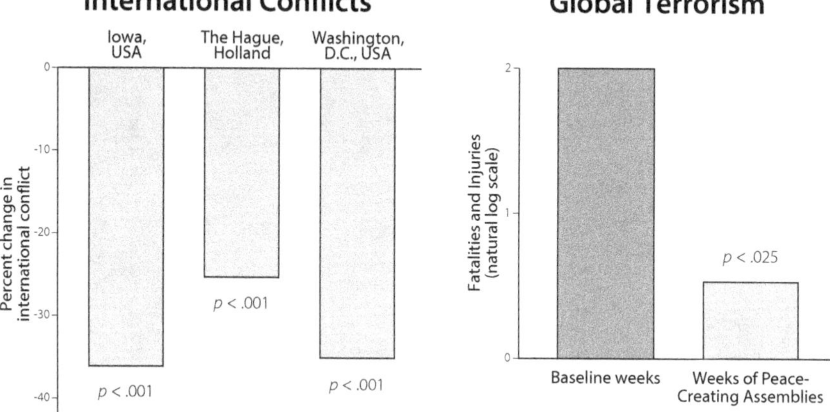

DECREASED WAR & TERRORISM

This study found that on the three occasions when World Peace Assemblies of people practicing the Transcendental Meditation (TM) and TM-Sidhi program, held in 1983–1984 at Maharishi International University in Iowa, in Holland, and in Washington, DC, approached the 7,000 threshold needed for global coherence, international conflicts decreased by more than 30%. In addition, international terrorism decreased by more than 70%.

International conflicts were assessed by content analysis of daily conflicts reported in *The New York Times* and *The London Times*. *The New York Times* has been widely used as the primary source for scoring international and civil conflicts. *The London Times* has a somewhat broader coverage of European and African events. Terrorism was assessed using data compiled by the Rand Corporation, whose data bank is derived from public domain sources by monitoring approximately 100 newspapers, journals, and periodicals.

The definition of terrorism used in compiling the database was "violence, or the threat of violence, calculated to create an atmosphere of fear and alarm." All events were international in scope, excluding domestic incidents. Terrorism during the three assemblies was aggregated and compared to a baseline of all other times when there was no assembly during the 2-year period.

The effects of the assemblies on international conflicts and terrorism were assessed by time series intervention analysis, which assesses the impact of the assembly independently from any cycles or trends in the data. This answers the question: Were the measured changes caused by the assembly, or could they have been predicted by existing trends?

When the coherence-creating group was large enough to have a predicted impact on increasing harmony in world consciousness, international conflicts decreased by 36%, 24%, and 35% respectively for the three assemblies, and that global terrorism decreased by 72% during the three assemblies combined, compared to the baseline period. The study ruled out the possibility that this reduction in terrorism was due to time of year, or to cycles, trends, or drifts in the measures used.

Reference. Orme-Johnson, D.W., Dillbeck, M.C., & Alexander, C.N (2003). Preventing terrorism and international conflict: Effects of large assemblies of participants in the Transcendental Meditation and TM-Sidhi programs. *Journal of Offender Rehabilitation*, 36, 283–302.

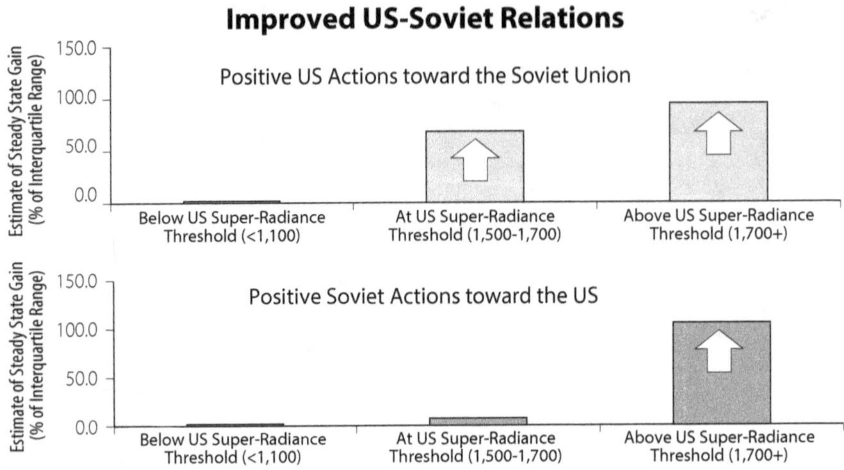

tm-077

MORE CORDIAL INTERNATIONAL RELATIONSHIPS

The most dramatic political change of the twentieth century is the warming of relations between the superpowers, with its enormous worldwide implications. This study was on the effects of a group practicing the Transcendental Meditation (TM) and TM-Sidhi program at Maharishi International University in Fairfield, Iowa, on US-Soviet relations. The study used data from the Zurich Project on East-West Relations, which tracked US-Soviet relations by content analysis of news events from 1979 to 1986.

At that time, the size of the group predicted to be large enough to affect the entire US (its Super-Radiance threshold of the square root of 1% of the population) was between 1,500-1700. The study found that when the group size reached the US Super-Radiance threshold, US relations toward the Soviets became more positive, but there was not yet an effect on the Soviets toward the US. Moreover, when the size of the group became even larger, over 1,700 TM and TM-Sidhi participants, the US actions toward the Soviets became even more positive and the Soviet actions toward the US also became significantly more positive.

This finding indicates that if we had a large enough permanent group of TM and TM-Sidhi participants that it would create perpetual world peace.

Reference: Gelderloos, P., Cavanaugh, K.L., & Davies, J.L. (1990). The dynamics of US-Soviet relations, 1979–1986: Effects of reducing social stress through the Transcendental Meditation and TM-Sidhi program. Paper presented at the Proceedings of the American Statistical Association, Alexandria, VA. Reprinted in *Collected papers,* Vol. 6, pp 4130-4137.

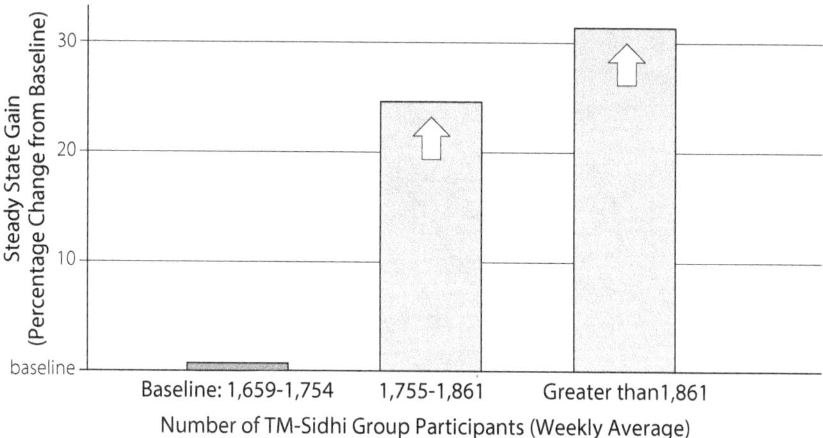

MORE POSITIVE, UPLIFTING ATTENTION

In 1984-1987, when the size of the Transcendental Meditation (TM) and TM-Sidhi group in the USA became large enough to have a predicted effect of increasing coherence in US national consciousness (1,755-1,861 participants), US president Ronald Reagan's statements about the Soviet Union became significantly more cordial. When the size of the group increased further to over 1,861 participants, the president's statements became even more positive. This suggests that increasing coherence in national consciousness caused the president to speak more positively.

Diagnostic tests and sensitivity analysis indicated that USSR president Gorbachev, pre-existing trends, seasonal or other cycles in Soviet behavior, or spurious regression could not explain the increased positivity of the statements of world leaders. Weekly fluctuations in the size of the TM-Sidhi group were random, eliminating many alternative explanations for the effect. For example, many political analysts regard the presidency of Gorbachev as responsible for the warming of US-Soviet relations. Yet President Gorbachev influenced the entire study period, which could not explain the specific times of increased positivity.

This study also found President Reagan made more positive statements about the USSR when the size of the coherence-creating group increased. This indicates that increased coherence in national consciousness increased the president's positivity and productivity in international relations.

President Reagan's statements about the Soviet Union were taken from the *Weekly Compilation of Presidential Documents*, published by the Office of the Federal Register of the National Archives.

Reference: Gelderloos, P., Cavanaugh, K.L., Frid, M.J., & Xue, X. (2019). Warming US-Soviet relations during the Cold War as measured by US presidential statements: Impact of the group practice of the Transcendental Meditation-Sidhi program. *Journal of Maharishi Vedic Research Institute, 9*, 93-134.

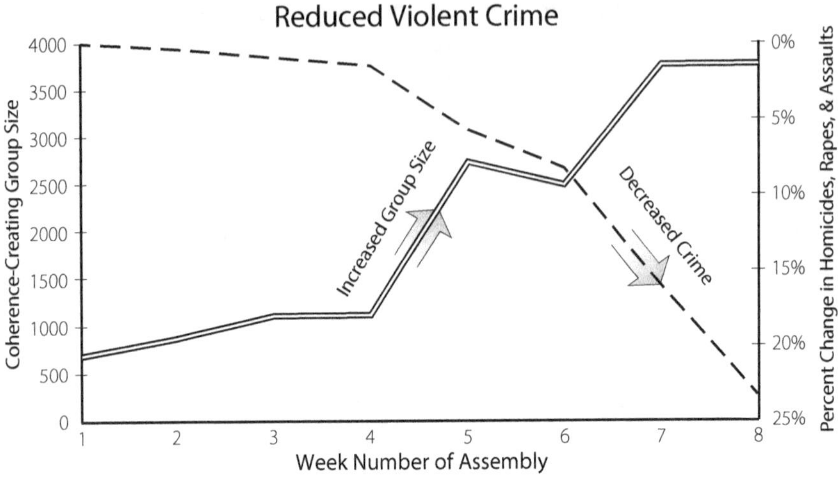

SAFER FROM VIOLENT CRIME

In the summer of 1993, 4000 advanced Transcendental Meditation (TM) and TM-Sidhi practitioners came to Washington, DC, USA for 53 consecutive days to be part of a Super-Radiance group demonstrating the Maharishi Effect.

The project predicted a 20% drop in crime, and notified the press in advance. A 27-member Project Review Board, comprising respected scientists, government leaders, and members of the District of Columbia Police Department, approved the research protocol—a time-series transfer function analysis of independent and dependent variables. The independent variable was the size of the Super-Radiance group between June 7 and July 30, which increased from approximately 1,000 to 4,000. The dependent variables were continuous daily or weekly crime data, extending before, during, and after the project. Other non-criminological indicators of social stress were also predicted to show improvement.

The chart above shows that as the size of the TM-Sidhi group increased (double line), violent crime decreased (dashed line). (Reference 1)

In a separate study, Goodman (1997) found that all such regularly reported sociological variables—accidental deaths, hospital emergency room trauma cases, emergency psychiatric calls, and complaints against police—improved significantly after the start of this Demonstration Project, in contrast to a trend of growing negativity prior to the projects. (Reference 2)

Reference 1: Hagelin, J.S., Rainforth, M.V., Orme-Johnson, D.W., Cavanaugh, K.L., Alexander, C.N., Shatkin, S.F., et al. Effects of group practice of the Transcendental Meditation program on preventing violent crime in Washington, DC: Results of the National Demonstration Project, June–July, 1993. *Social Indicators Research.* 1999; 47(2):153–201.

Reference 2: Goodman, R., Orme-Johnson, D.W., Rainforth, M.V., and Goodman, D., Transforming Political Institutions through Individual and Collective Consciousness: the Maharishi Effect in government, *Proceedings of the 1997 Annual Meeting of the American Political Science Association*, Washington, DC, August 28-31, 1997.

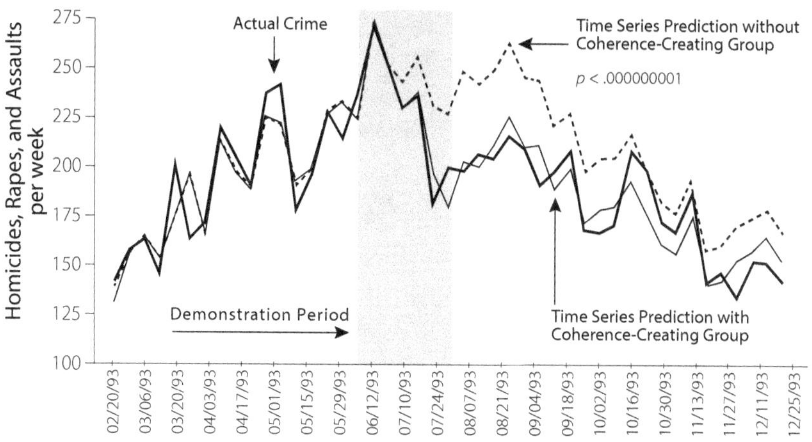

SAFER, HAPPIER COMMUNITIES

During the Washington DC Demonstration Project in the summer of 1993, time-series analysis was also used to model actual crime levels with the Transcendental Meditation (TM) and TM-Sidhi program Super-Radiance group, versus predicted crime levels without the group. When the group was largest, actual violent crime had dropped more than 23% (p < .000000001) below the level predicted without the Super-Radiance group, one chance in one billion that the effect was due to chance.

A second finding of the Washington, DC Demonstration Project compared predicted crime rates with and without the Super-Radiance group.

Analysis of 41 previous studies had predicted reduced crime when the group reached a particular size.

In this project, crime decreased more than 32% (p = .00008).

Extensive additional time-series analysis could identify no other explanations to account for this drop in crime, including temperature, precipitation, changes in police surveillance, weekend effects, or trends in the data.

Reference: Hagelin, J.S., Rainforth, M.V., Orme-Johnson, D.W., Cavanaugh, K.L., Alexander, C.N., Shatkin, S.F., et al. Effects of group practice of the Transcendental Meditation program on preventing violent crime in Washington DC: Results of the National Demonstration Project, June–July, 1993. *Social Indicators Research*. 1999; 47(2):153–201.

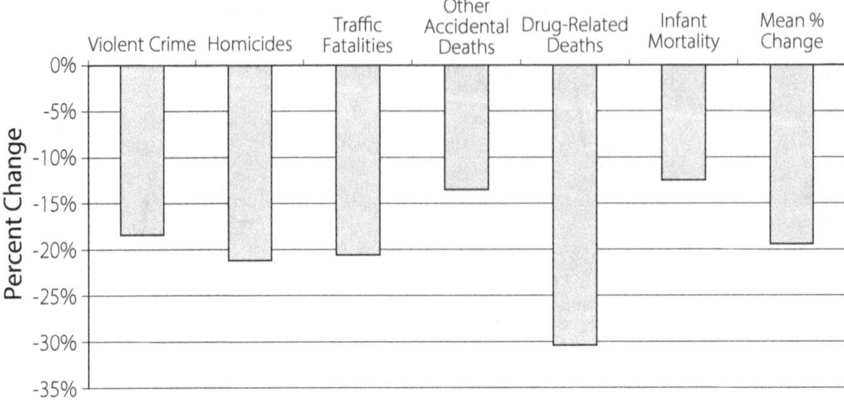

√1% GROUP CREATES A BETTER LIFE

During a four-year period from 2007 to 2010, a group of the √1% of the US population (approximately 1,725 at the time) practiced the Transcendental Meditation (TM) and TM-Sidhi program, including Yogic Flying, together at Maharishi International University in Fairfield, Iowa, creating a powerful influence of coherence in the nation. The chart above shows the percent changes in crime and fatalities in the USA for 2007 to 2010 compared to trends during the baseline period 2002 through 2006: • violent crime, -18%, • murder, -21.2%, • traffic fatalities, -20.6% • other accidental fatalities, -13.5%, • drug-related deaths, -30.4%, • infant mortality, -12.5%.

On average, there was a 19.1% reduction in rates of fatalities of the six variables. (References 1–4)

Reference 1: Dillbeck, M.C., & Cavanaugh, K.L. (2016). Societal violence and collective consciousness: Reduction of US homicide and urban violent crime rates. *SAGE Open,* April-June, 1–16.

Reference 2: Cavanaugh, K.L., & Dillbeck, M.C. (2017). The contribution of proposed field effects of consciousness to the prevention of US accidental fatalities: Theory and empirical tests. *Journal of Consciousness Studies,* 24(1-2), 53–86

Reference 3: Dillbeck, M.C., & Cavanaugh, K.L. (2017). Group Practice of the Transcendental Meditation and TM-Sidhi Program and Reductions in Infant Mortality and Drug-Related Death: A Quasi-Experimental Analysis. *SAGE Open,* January-March, 1–15.

Reference 4: Cavanaugh, K.L., & Dillbeck, M.C. (2017). Field Effects of Consciousness and Reduction in US Urban Murder Rates: Evaluation of a Prospective Quasi-Experiment. *Journal of Health and Environmental Research,* 3(3-1), 32–43

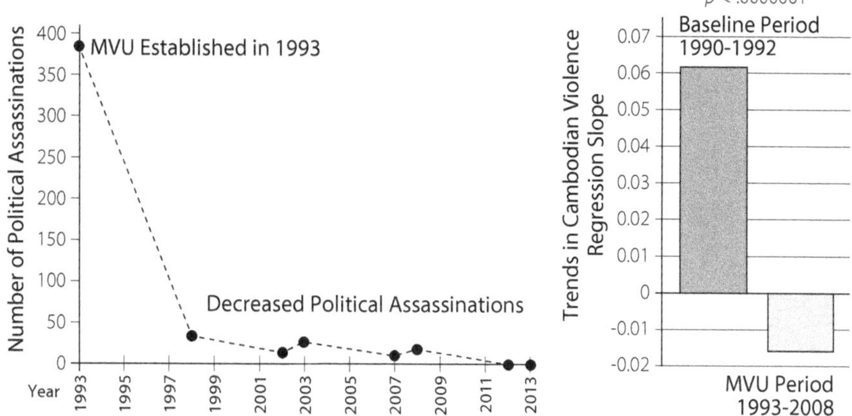

MORE STABLE POLITICS & SOCIETY

In Cambodia, the combined effects of individual Transcendental Meditation (TM) practice, and group practice of the TM Sidhi program, accumulated over the years to reduce socio-political violence.

The left chart shows significantly declining socio-political violence in Cambodia in 1993, after Maharishi Vedic University (MVU) established group practice of the TM & TM-Sidhi program by enough people to affect life in Cambodia. Political killings decreased sharply from 380 in 1993 to 40 by 1998, with a steady decline to 23 in 2008 and to zero in 2013.

The right chart documents a comprehensive monthly automated content analysis of violent acts such as riots, armed attacks, battles, assassinations, coups, bombings, and violent crowd control. It shows that a rising trend of violence in Cambodia during the baseline period of 1990 to 1992 (dark bar) transformed into a trend of decreasing violence (light bar), which started in 1993, when group practice of the TM & TM-Sidhi practice was established.

This reversal in the rising baseline trend of violence was large and highly statistically significant ($p < 1 \times 10^{-7}$, or less than one chance in 10 million). Contrary to existing trends and community expectations, the shift to a steadily declining trend of violence began in January 1993 with the onset of group practice of TM and the TM-Sidhi program at Maharishi Vedic University in Cambodia. For the 16 years group practice was in operation, the total decline in socio-political violence was 96.2% (6% per year) relative to the end of the baseline period.

References: Fergusson, L.C., & Cavanaugh, K.L. (2019). Socio-political violence in Cambodia between 1990 and 2008: An explanatory mixed methods study of social coherence. *Studies in Asian Social Science*, 6(2), 1-45.

Fergusson, L.C. (2016). The impact of Maharishi Vedic University on Cambodian economic and social indicators from 1980 to 2015. *Journal of Maharishi Vedic Research Institute*, 2, 77-135.

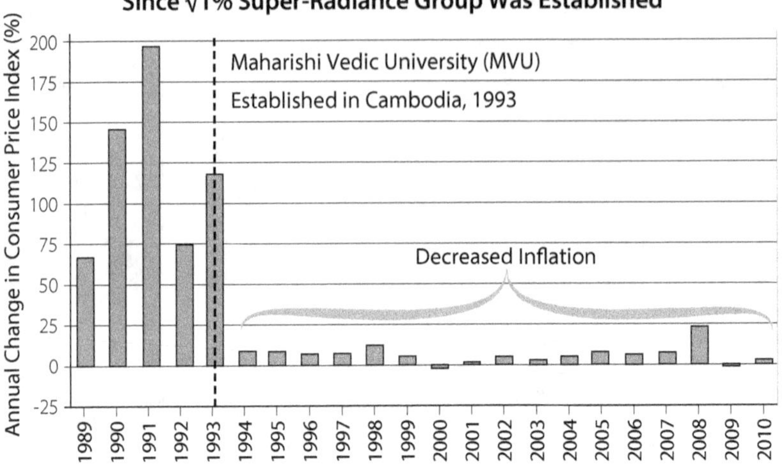

LESS INFLATION

The chart above shows that with increased national coherence created by the establishment of a Super-Radiance group at MVU in 1993, the consumer price index dropped sharply, indicating reduced inflation. Reduced inflation means slower increase in the cost of a basket of goods and services consumed by households.

In this atmosphere of increased economic stability, Cambodia's economy took off. The percent change in purchasing power of its gross national income (a measure of domestic and foreign earnings by Cambodians) was 190% compared to lesser change among other nations in the surrounding area: Thailand, Lao PDR, and Vietnam.

Reference: Fergusson, L. (2016). Vedic Science-based education, poverty removal and social wellbeing: A case history of Cambodia from 1980 to 2015. *Journal of Indian Education*, 41(4), 16–45.

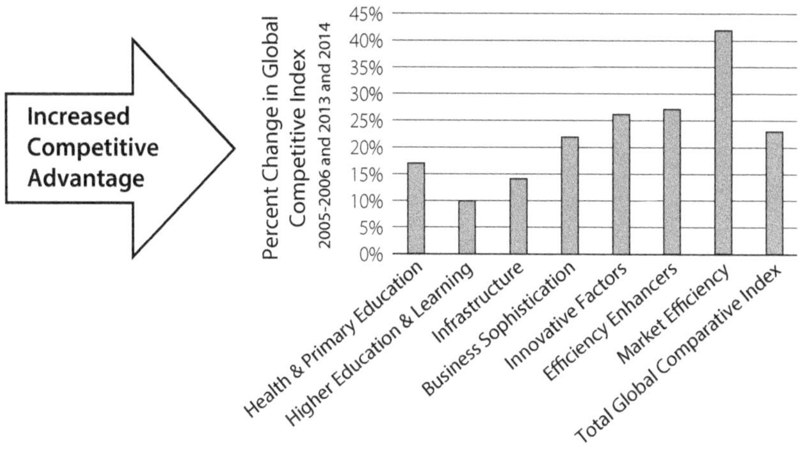

STRONGER ECONOMY

The chart above showed Cambodia's gains on the Global Competitive Index, which compares its growth with 144 other countries. Cambodia gained 10 to 15 percentile points on education and infrastructure and 20 to 27 percentile points on business sophistication, innovation, and efficiency enhancers, such as education and training. This translated into remarkable 42% gains in market efficiency, which reflects intelligent awareness of market trends and creative positioning of one's products and services to supply emerging market needs. Cambodia is a model of how creating a Super-Radiance group in a country can create economic stability, and foster the blossoming of national creativity. (Reference 1)

Nine years later, in a study from 2002–2015, of the poorest countries in the world, Cambodia led other developing nations in achieving 90% or more success on reaching the 2015 targets for reducing poverty, undernourishment, and infant and maternal mortality, as well as improving access to clean water, and enrollment in primary education. The World Bank commented of Cambodia, "Where have all the poor gone?" (Reference 2)

Reference 1: Fergusson, L. (2016). The impact of Maharishi Vedic University on Cambodian economic and social indicators from 1980 to 2015. *Journal of Maharishi Vedic Research Institute, 2*, 77–135.

Fergusson, L. (2016). Vedic Science-based education, poverty removal and social wellbeing: A case history of Cambodia from 1980 to 2015. *Journal of Indian Education*, 41(4), 16–45.

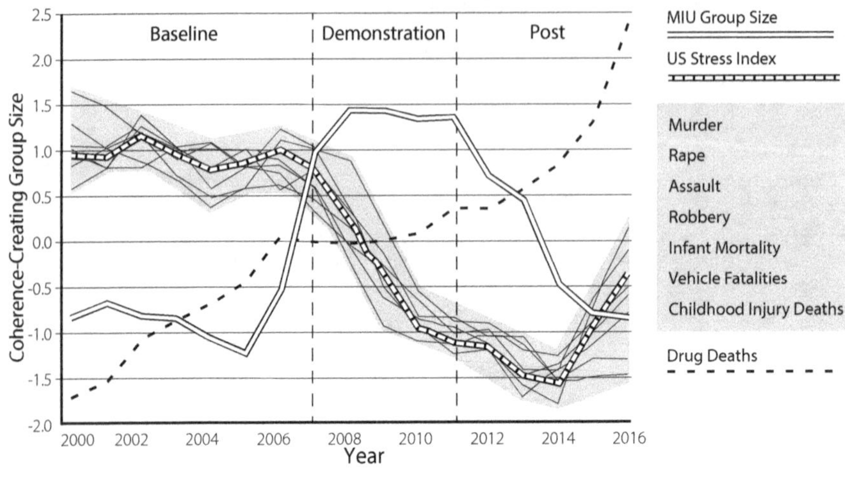

tm-085

SUFFERING VARIES WITH SUPER-RADIANCE SIZE

This study found that when a group in Iowa, USA practicing the Transcendental Meditation (TM) and TM-Sidhi program reached the predicted √1% of the US population, there was a *simultaneous* decrease in the trends of multiple national stress indicators: murder, rape, assault, robbery, infant mortality, vehicle fatalities, and childhood and adolescent deaths by injuries. The rapid rise of deaths from drug overdose slowed significantly during the demonstration period. When the group size dropped, the change in all stress indicators slowed and then turned around and started increasing again.

The study analyzed all factors known to influence the indices of national stress and found that none could explain the reduction in the individual variables, much less the simultaneous reduction in all of them at the predicted time. In fact, the observed reductions in crime were in the opposite direction of what was widely predicted to happen due to the high level of unemployment and low level of incarceration at the time.

This study also showed that the negative trends began to rise again when the size of the coherence-creating group decreased (2012–2016). For example, the precipitous drop in size of the group (2013–2014) corresponded with a rapid increase in negative trends. Clearly the urgent responsibility of our time is to create and maintain coherence-creating Super-Radiance groups for every nation.

References: Orme-Johnson, D.W., Cavanaugh, K.L., Dillbeck, M.C., & Goodman, R.S. (2022). Field-Effects of Consciousness: A Seventeen-Year Study of the Effects of Group Practice of the Transcendental Meditation and TM-Sidhi Programs on reducing national stress in the United States. *World Journal of Social Science*, 19(1).

Cavanaugh, K.L., Dillbeck, M.C., & Orme-Johnson, D.W. (2022). Evaluating a Field Theory of Consciousness and Social Change: Group Practice of Transcendental Meditation and Homicide Trends. *Studies in Asian Social Science*, 8(1), 1-32.

Dillbeck, M.C., & Cavanaugh, K.L. (2023). Empirical Evaluation of the Possible Contribution of Group Practice of the Transcendental Meditation and TM-Sidhi Program to Reduction in Drug-Related Mortality. *Medicina*, 59, 1-32.

> *To find the TM center near you, go to*
> TM.org/Choose-your-country

For More Information

The TM Book further explorations
   TheTMbook.com

Maharishi International University
   MIU.edu

Global Country of World Peace
   GlobalCountry.org

Dr. Tony Nader
   DrTonyNader.com

Global Union of Scientists for Peace
   GUSP.org

TM for Women
   TM-Women.org & TM-Nurses.org

Maharishi Vastu Architecture
   MaharishiVastu.org

Maharishi AyurVeda
   MIU.edu/AyurVeda

TM Research Discussion
   TruthAboutTM.org

About the Authors

David W. Orme-Johnson holds an AB in psychology from Columbia University (1963) and MA and PhD in Psychology from the University of Maryland (1965, 1969). He is Professor Emeritus of Psychology at Maharishi International University, where he was a founding faculty in 1972, serving as chair of the psychology department and director of its doctoral program. Dr. Orme-Johnson has authored more than 100 publications on the effects of the Transcendental Meditation technique, having pioneered in its effects on stress reduction, prison rehabilitation, health, neurophysiological effects, cognitive abilities, on creating coherence in collective consciousness to improve the quality of life in society, and world peace.

Denise Denniston Gerace became a teacher of the TM program in 1971. She has taught TM in Omaha, Nebraska; Los Angeles, California; New York City; and Tucson, Arizona, as well as working at the United States national headquarters for TM, and at the International Capital of the Age of Enlightenment in Europe. She holds a BA in English Literature and Art History from the University of Arizona (1969) and an MA and PhD in Philosophy of Education from the University of California at Berkeley (1980, 1988). She is Emeritus Faculty of the Science of Creative Intelligence at Maharishi International University and past Co-Principal of the Maharishi School Middle and Upper Schools.

Chart Headlines, *alphabetical*

Chart Titles, *alphabetical*

Publications Cited

Topic List